YOU AND YOUR EYES

Lawrence Lewison

Second Edition, Revised and Enlarged

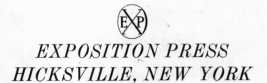

EXPOSITION PRESS
HICKSVILLE, NEW YORK

Second Edition, Revised

Copyright © 1960, 1978 by Lawrence Lewison

Library of Congress Catalog Card Number: 77-80595

ISBN 0-682-48926-3

Printed in the United States of America

Contents

Acknowledgment

For permission to quote from material, some of it published, some unpublished, thanks are expressed to the following:

American Optical Co., Southbridge, Mass.
Bausch & Lomb Optical Co., Rochester, N.Y.
Contact Lens Specialists, New York, N.Y.
Kollmorgen Optical Co., Northampton, Mass.
Titmus Optical Co., Petersburg, Va.
Vent-Air Contact Lens Laboratories, New York, N.Y.

You and Your Eyes

Introduction

As you read this, the printed markings on this page form tiny images on the back of your eyes. Letters become words, words blend into sentences, sentences shape thoughts and ideas.

Impressions and responses are conveyed and awakened in your brain almost instantaneously, the result of a complex coordination of optical stimuli and nerve impulse.

The telling of this optical and nerve partnership is the story of your eyes. It is a fascinating one—with obscure beginnings, an engrossing plot, and an ending still to be written.

Its chief character is the most precious of the five senses—our eyesight. For complete participation in the joy of living as well as in our ordinary day-to-day activities the means by which we see—our eyes—are unquestionably one of man's most cherished possessions.

Our story's chief villains are the defects to which our eyes are subject. They cause this print to be blurred or distorted, they require this page to be held uncomfortably close or awkwardly far, they mean distant objects are indistinguishable or indistinct. They lead as well to eye-aches and eye-inflammations, to headaches and tiredness, to boredom and even emotional disturbances.

These defects are the so-called refractive anomalies, which sometimes are and sometimes are not correctable by what we know as eyeglasses. They account for 75 to 85% of all eye difficulties and afflict more than 60% of the world's population.

Its hero is science's never-ending search for means to avert, correct, neutralize, remedy and eliminate these defects . . . its plot— the early, groping efforts to utilize naturally-occurring crystals and primitive potions, the awakening use of painstakingly-fabricated glasses and medieval lotions, and modern-day's medical, surgical, psychological and optical therapies. For in today's resources for visual correction are methods and devices barely dreamed of short decades ago.

The story we tell is not a simple one.

It must trace its way through the development of the eye, the causes of its many malfunctions, the correction of its inadequacies by historic means including eyeglasses, and arrive at the consideration of the most modern means available. Throughout, it will strive to explore and evaluate how these means originated, their rationale and effectiveness.

In one direction our inquiry will culminate in what we know as "contact lenses"—those tiny bits of plastic which seem so miraculous. Their emergence upon the scene in current years has had tremendous impact. What are these modern lenses? When are they used? What are their pros and cons? These are among the questions we will seek to answer.

Finally, we will venture some predictions as to the future of eyesight correction. What will the human eye be like in years to come? What defects, now unknown, may appear? What remedies now in use may be discarded? What new means of correction, now undreamed of, may develop? What advances are virtual certainties within the next half-century?

All of this our story will try to tell.

If it acquaints the reader with modern means of eyesight correction, if it broadens his understanding that, for one thing, eyeglasses are not the only way to correct defective vision, it will more than serve its purpose.

I

Are Glasses Still Necessary?

For centuries the problem of defective sight has burdened mankind.

For years eyeglasses, the two circles of glass perched and supported in position in front of the eyes, have been considered the dominant means of correcting this troubled vision.

The person who did not see as well as his neighbor would turn to eyeglasses. The one who had to strain and frown and squint, the one who suffered headaches and whose eyes tired, turned to glasses. And those whom glasses did not help were virtually abandoned to a life of discomfort or sightlessness.

Is this still true?

Modern science says no. And well over six million Americans, together with countless others all over the world, agree. Their defective, troubled sight has been corrected by other means.

Through the miracle of new discoveries with regard to the nature of vision, through the research and development which led to drug therapy, visual exercises and contact lenses, these millions have been able to gain corrected and comfortable sight without glasses. They have been able to advance beyond the limitations, handicaps, and even frustrations which, it has been found, glasses impose on many wearers.

The miracle that was wrought came about when the same science which labored to perfect eyeglasses also worked to achieve something better—something which served to replace glasses and which also restored vision when glasses did not. It achieved this

13

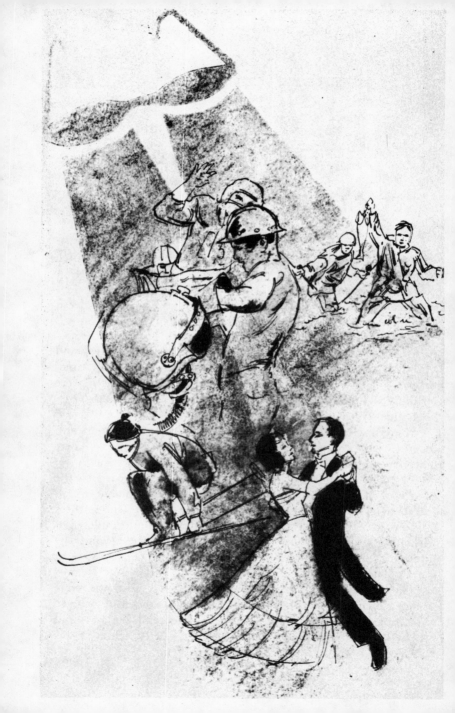

in the form of advanced therapy, special vision-training exercises and modern-day invisible contact lenses. It brought the day closer when glasses would be used only as a *first* resort, and then only by those who, for one reason or another, could not avail themselves immediately of one of these new remedies.

Despite the fact that the number of eyeglass wearers increases daily as better methods are utilized to uncover eye defects—there are some 75 million eyeglass-wearing Americans today—more and more will the new sufferer from poor or uncomfortable vision walk a newer, brighter path to corrected sight.

Aside from the eye condition which ordinary glasses cannot correct, and apart from the physical and optical disadvantages of regular eyeglasses, there were still other reasons why research did not pause in its quest for a better solution to the problem of eye correction.

Only studies allied to modern psychology could have provided those reasons. And they did. Studies completed only a year or two ago uncovered the motivation that would not let this research die.

Man's desire to be rid of glasses—to present a normal, un-handicapped appearance to the outside world, was found to be deep-rooted and intense. The psychological trauma created in the eyeglass wearer, though long suspected, was never so clearly understood as in recent years.

Whether or not it was the post-war era which did it, or whether these recent years simply permitted their expression more openly, the fact was that whole new sets of unsatisfied needs were revealed in these studies.

Foremost among them was the desire for physical and social improvement. The modern man (and woman) is no longer willing to accept physical defects which may be a roadblock on the path to improved social relationships and increased business opportunities. For one thing, eyeglasses are a glaring sign of a physical defect; this explains why they have always been and remain a prime target for elimination.

Specifically, these studies revealed that job opportunities and chances for advancement in the business world increased as obvious physical handicaps were less in evidence. Subconsciously, there was a barrier imposed between the eyeglass wearer—particularly the wearer of strong glasses, and the personnel man who determined his chances of promotion. All other things being equal, the choice was usually in favor of the unencumbered individual . . . the one who *didn't* wear glasses!

In a host of modern-day occupations too, eyeglasses are found to be a distinct physical hazard. Breakage, the effect of exposure to weather and temperature changes, high-speed transportation requiring quick eye movements—all these make glasses unsuitable for many types of conditions. Working within constricted areas—mines, underwater, inside helmets—likewise illustrates the impracticality of glasses. Physically cramped quarters make mechanical and plumbing repairs, for instance, doubly difficult by anyone wearing glasses.

Heightened sports-consciousness—the direct outgrowth of increased leisure stemming from the improved living standards generated by the war and post-war years—this too has influenced the motivation to be free of glasses.

During the course of industrial and government surveys occasioned by the war effort, safety engineers pinpointed eyeglasses as a likely cause of accidents and of many serious injuries suffered in athletic and automobile, as well as industrial mishaps.

All these factors seemed to come into sharp focus during the post-war years and when coupled with the strongest motivation of all—the desire to be attractive, the force was an impelling one.

Glasses were and still are stigmatized in word and thought. At best they have been tolerated and despite attempts to make them chic and becoming, have never been accepted as desirable adjuncts to good grooming and good appearance.

Propelled by this force research kept on apace. Programs originating during the war years continued in motion, seeking ways to eliminate or at least reduce the need for glasses.

They have borne fruit. Modern science can now point to at least four means of reducing, if not wholly eliminating, the need for glasses as corrective measures.

Science has found that approximately 5 to 10% of the eyeglass-wearing population could be relieved of wearing glasses with proper remedial measures in living and working conditions, both physical and psychological.

Approximately 2 to 5% could be cured of existing eye conditions through proper diet and the use of drugs and medication.

Approximately 10 to 15% could be spared the need to wear glasses by the proper application of eye exercises or what is called visual training.

Approximately 70 to 80% could eliminate glasses by changing to modern contact lenses.

Of these categories the first two are not unexpected advances in general ophthalmological science: new standards of nutrition and environment, new findings in therapy and prevention, and the greatly accentuated emphasis on psychology, both normal and abnormal, as applied to vision, viz. remedial reading.

Visual training and modern contact lenses as a substitute means of sight correction—as well as a corrective means where glasses could not serve—however, are relatively new. Their currently successful application is almost a direct result of intensified research specifically conceived during the war years. Many candidates for military service, for one thing, both here and abroad emphasized the need for this research effort. In large measure they are to thank for the strides made since the war.

For these strides pointed out without question that in many, many cases, glasses are truly not necessary.

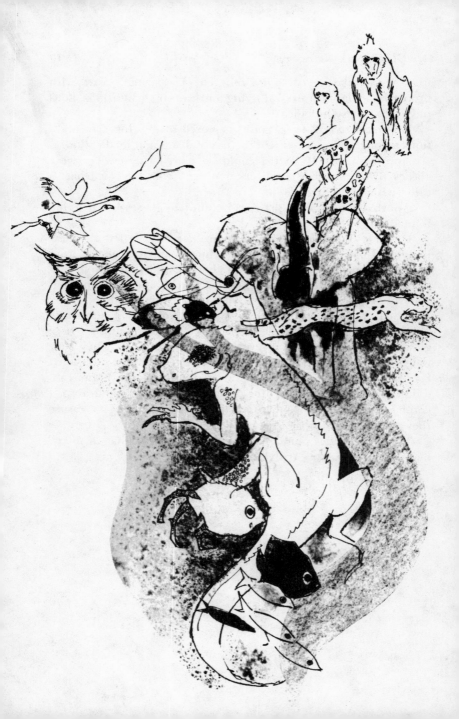

II

The Eye—
Then and Now

Was pre-historic man stronger and healthier than the present-day human being? ｜

Could primitive man see as well as modern man? Did he use any implements to correct poor eyesight?

How did eyesight affect the survival of man years ago?

What was the human eye like centuries ago? How did his eyesight serve his basic needs?

Our eyes and our general health are actually in far better condition today than ever before in man's history. The toll which systemic conditions and degenerative diseases exact of the eye is more widely understood and consequently better controlled than ever before. With advances in personal hygiene and public health, many dread eye diseases have been virtually eliminated. The proper importance attached to nutrition and lighting enables the human eye of today to be healthier and less prone to disease than at any time in the past.

Nevertheless, the role of evolution must not be overlooked. Here is where the problem arises, for the human eye of today has not evolved fast enough to keep pace with the exacting and unique demands of modern living. Problems and tasks the eye must face today are not the same as those of prehistoric or even historic times.

The eye originally developed in its primordial state as a tool of perception—one of several used essentially for the purpose of survival. In the course of its evolution and its adaptation to man's needs, the eye enabled him to defend himself, to hunt, to fish, and to function as a prime aid in the battle for survival and mastery of his environment.

Today the eye serves more complicated and intricate needs— needs greatly in advance, in many cases, of its comparatively simple structure.

If we study the evolution of the eye we can observe how it changed from a rudimentary pigmented area sensitive to light and heat to the specialized organ it is today. As the processes of evolution unfold there is little doubt that the human eye of the distant tomorrow will adapt itself better to the visual needs of the civilization of the future. Indeed, it may bear little resemblance to the eye of today.

But, to begin at the beginning, how did the eye originate?

The origin of the eye is linked to the nature of light itself. And the story of light is in reality the story of life. For light— the visible radiant energy emanating from the sun—is the very foundation of life. Without photosynthesis—the light process which converts water and carbon dioxide into the organic substances which are the bases for all living things, life as we know it would never have come into being.

Photosynthesis—the basic light-controlled chemical reaction characterizing the vegetable world—is without question light's greatest contribution to nature's scheme. Yet light also serves other purposes. It produces other profound chemical changes—

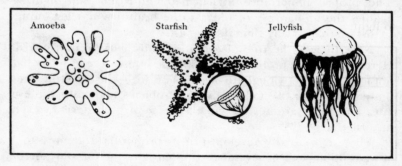

Amoeba   Starfish   Jellyfish

Fig. 4: Primitive forms of life react to both light and heat.

so-called "photo-chemical" reactions—of great variety and effect on living organisms.

In simple creatures, such as the lowly amoeba, the chemical reaction produced by the impact of light liberates energy, causing a change in general activity. The amoeba is all eye, for any part on which light impinges will draw away from it. Even when the amoeba divides, each part will respond in the same way.

This withdrawal is the same effect caused by other, more direct stimuli—mechanical, chemical, thermal or electrical.

With other such organisms light may induce a change in form such as contraction. There may be lessened activity in the presence of light in some cases, and increased activity in others. Certainly there is almost always an awareness of light as distinguished from dark. The very periodicity of light and dark, day and night, has had its far-reaching effect on the activities and habits of living things, indeed on the whole scheme of both animal and vegetable life, from time immemorial.

In an evolutionary sense light has also had pronounced effect on the structure of animal tissue, causing the origin and the development of the eye. Originally there were specially differentiated areas pigmented for the greater absorption of light—either to utilize its energy or to protect against its excess.

These simple eye-spots or pigment-spots were sensitive both to heat and light and in some cases projected somewhat beyond the surface of the animal's body. With the passage of time this spot lost its sensitivity to heat and became more highly sensitive to light.

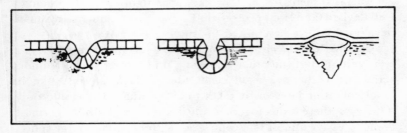

Fig. 5: The pigment-spot invaginates and becomes a dimple-eye.

Nature further provided—in more favored organisms—some protection to this sensitive spot. It receded into a depressed area, at the bottom of a pit. The starfish is an example of this type of dimple eye. The spot could then be protected against glancing side blows.

There still was no way to prevent sand from entering and injuring the pigment. The next step was to cover the opening of the pit by a transparent layer of skin. This protected the precious pigment area from dangerous objects and sand. Mucous —which nature had formerly supplied in front of the pigment spot, was now enclosed, and began to coalesce and form the internal structures of the eye we know today. An external mucous flow came into being to prevent external objects from remaining on the eye's surface.

And as evolution continued its endless process of selection and survival, we began to get a practical instrument for reproducing light images by optical means on sensitive receptor cells—not just the sensation of light.

This meant that an actual lens system (which we will describe later) was evolved that refracted or focused the light rays entering the eye, producing an image on the back of the eye. These miniature images—identical with those produced by inanimate means, were registered on what was formerly just a pigment spot but which now became a highly complex system of nerve endings. These nerve endings conveyed the image to a central nervous organ—eventually the brain, which in turn permitted the creature thus stimulated to identify the image with its source.

An instrument for what we know as sight came into being— well-devised and well-protected. Each creature, including man, developed an eye best suited for the life it was to lead.

Certain fish developed two focusing arrangements—one for seeing in air and the other for seeing under water. The flounder starts life with an eye on each side of its head, just like its neighbors, but later on it takes to swimming on one side only. The eyes then grow together until they are both uppermost. Some fish have almost telescopic eyes, with unusually large spherical lenses concentrating light rays on an extremely small area, producing high brightness.

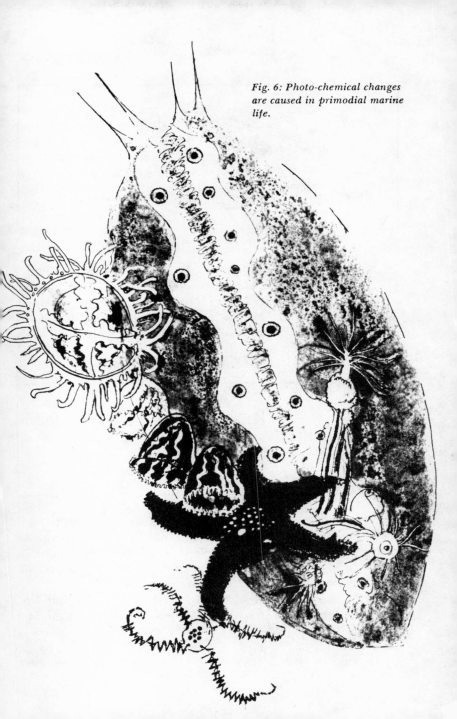

Fig. 6: Photo-chemical changes are caused in primodial marine life.

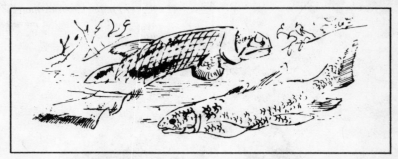

Fig. 7: Fish develop special eye structures and lenses.

In the case of insects, for example, two types of eyes evolved—compound and simple. The fly, the bee, the moth, the mosquito, and other such creatures have two compound eyes, one on either side of the head, in addition to a number of simple eyes. Each compound eye is composed of at least six and as many as 28,000 small eyes set in tubular facets, each tube leading to a bit of pigment connected to the central nervous system.

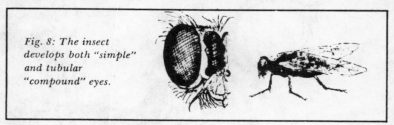

Fig. 8: The insect develops both "simple" and tubular "compound" eyes.

At the top of each tube there is a lens which throws its own tiny image of a small part of its surroundings on its particular pigment spot, so that a complete mosaic picture is formed in much the same manner as the dots of a photographic screen are combined to form a complete picture of an object.

The simple insect eye, together with the compound eye, evidently serves to perceive near objects as well as light and darkness, while it is believed that the compound eye also sees motion and distant objects.

In animals with a backbone—the vertebrates, the eye more

closely approaches our own. A quasi-spherical, almost egg-shaped body, it has the following properties: a transparent front surface highly curved to act as a strong, light-focusing lens (the cornea); an expansile and contractile membrane acting as a diaphragm to control the amount of entering light (the iris); an opening within this diaphragm (the pupil); a lens suspended behind this pupil serving as an accessory focusing agent (the crystalline lens); and a specialized neural membrane serving as the plate on which light images are focused (the retina).

As evolution proceeded, muscles were developed both inside and outside the eye chamber. Inside muscles served to control the focusing of the crystalline lens and the changing of size of the pupil; outside muscles controlled and directed the movements of the eye—at first independently and later on in unison with its mate.

Tear glands and ducts had their origin when the amphibia—animals at home either on land or sea (the frog, the crocodile, etc.), appeared on the scene. Here a built-in lubrication system for washing and moistening the eye became important. In the case of the frog, it is curious to note, its lower lid winks upward whereas in higher levels of life the upper lid winks downward.

Birds are unique in two respects. First, their eyes change focus by altering the curvature of the corneal or front surface of the eye rather than changing the curvature of the inside crystalline lens surface. Second, birds can barely move their eyeballs and depend on head movements to see in different directions.

Nevertheless, some birds have extremely sharp vision, and the term eagle-eyed is very apropos. The eyes of wild birds are invariably what we call farsighted (better able to see distant objects); while domesticated species, poultry, parrots, etc., tend to become nearsighted (better able to see near objects), astigmatic (unequal focusing power), or both, and develop eye diseases more readily. The same is true of wild animals as contrasted with domesticated species— (a valuable clue as to the effect of present-day domesticating civilization on the eyes of man).

Wild animals too (and this was carried forward to their tame

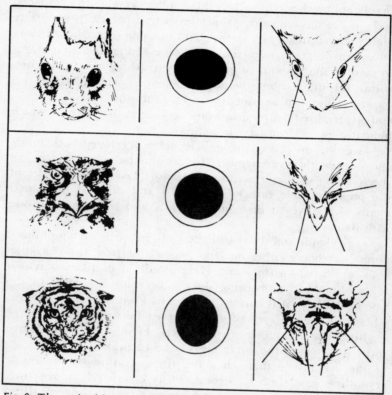

Fig. 9: The squirrel has a horizontal pupil and excellent panoramic vision. The eagle has a round pupil and extremely acute forward vision. The tiger has a vertical pupil and a full front field of vision.

brothers) developed characteristic advantages as aids to survival. Vertical pupil slits rather than round ones are present in animals who live primarily on a vertical plane and must climb and jump to avoid or initiate attack (tigers, cats, etc.). Horizontal pupil slits are the rule for animals who rely on speed for escape or feed on a horizontal plane (horses, deer, etc.).

Differences in eye size—as related to body size—also developed under the press of circumstance and necessity. Large eyes with large fields of vision developed for fast-moving creatures—the horse, the eagle, the ostrich, the shark, and the eyes are nearly twice the size of man's. Small eyes developed for slow-moving animals such as the reptiles.

On all levels, however, we notice the fundamental similarity of the eye and the fact that it is virtually identical in all higher animals including man. The eyeball is an almost spherical body enclosed in a bony cavity at the front of the skull—partially surrounded by eyelids, tear glands, ducts, muscles, blood vessels and nerves.

In addition, among the very highest animals—the Primates which include man and monkeys, we find without exception that the eyes were placed so that they are directed forward in a single gaze at a distant object. This subsequently gives rise to the exercise of convergence, where both eyes turn together to focus on a near object.

Binocular vision in all its aspects first made its appearance in the Primates, and gave rise to difficulties which contribute much to our story.

Further, man and the monkeys alone have a central fixation area or macula—where acute vision is surrounded by areas of gradually diminishing acuity. To be more explicit, it is in the Primates that an area was especially reserved and sensitive to the differentiation of form and outline, over and above the customary sensitivity to light and motion. Lower down in the evolutionary scale only this latter sensitivity is present, and as we ascend, this sensitivity becomes more and more the function of the peripheral parts of the retina.

Consequently, in the Primates the central macula has lost some of this sensitivity and only the periphery is highly sensitive to light. It is for this reason that a dim object is better viewed obliquely. Its image is cast on the peripheral areas composed mostly of rods—the primitive nerve elements more sensitive to light and therefore adapted to dim or nocturnal vision. It would be more accurate to say the central macular area is composed of advanced nerve elements—the cones, which have progressed beyond the rods and become perceptive to form and outline, sacrificing, as a result, some of their sensitivity to light and motion.

In animals below the level of monkeys, divergence of the eyes (turning away from each other), becomes greater as the evolutionary scale is descended. In the case of rodents, reptiles, amphibia and fish the eyes are at opposite sides of the head. In many cases such animals see better to the rear than to the front, and in these creatures there is no central macula. In some there is a particularly sensitive strip of conelike elements which spreads horizontally along the back of the eye (particularly in the higher mammals), so that even though acute central form vision is absent they have the advantage of a larger area of relatively good form vision.

Birds, most reptiles and some mammals have three eyelids. Most fish and some reptiles have no lids at all, with the eye covered simply by transparent skin. Again, this is closely related to their place in the evolutionary scale.

Color vision seems to be more extensively developed in man than in other forms of life. This is probably due to the different coloring matter in the pigment layer along the back of the eye and also to the specialized development of "cone" vision. In man the coloring matter is purple; in other animals it could be yellow, orange or green. But whatever the color, it fades under the stimulus of light (the so-called "bleaching" action on the visual purple) and this becomes the trigger action of nervous impulses which give rise to the sensation of sight. In this bleaching action too, we notice a basic factor common to all eyes.

Encased on the front by the highly polished corneal surface and on the rear by the pigment layer spotted with rods and cones, all the inner structures of this remarkable organ ultimately became suspended in a viscous, gel-like medium. In its anterior portion—between the cornea and the crystalline lens, this medium is called the "aqueous" humor, because of its close resemblance to pure water. In its posterior portion—between the lens and the retina, the name "vitreous" humor is applied, because of its greater resemblance to a glass-like substance.

Throughout there is an analogy between the eye and a camera —with the highly-polished transparent cornea as the front lens accounting for more than 80% of the total refracting power of the

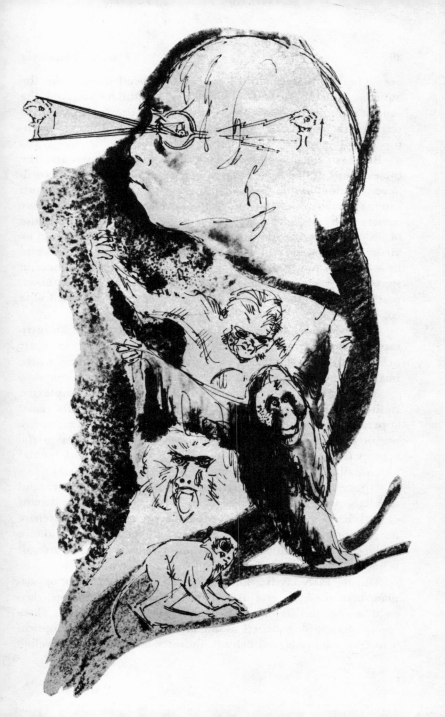

eye. The adjustable multi-focus lens suspended between the aqueous and the vitreous accounts for the difference. And the camera's photographic plate is usurped by the highly-sensitive retina with its rod and cone nerve endings as individual receptors.

But here the resemblance between the human eye and the camera ends. True, each receives images upside down in accordance with immutable laws of optics. Each has a lining to absorb internal reflections. But until the arrival of the modern-day camera with its electronic diaphragm, the eye was unique because of its self-adjusting pupillary opening. It remains unique by virtue of its curved receiving plate—rather than the flat one found in a camera—and by combining, in one neat little instrument, a stereoscopic movie camera, developer, projector, filing cabinet, precision range-finder and depth perceptor, all in true-to-life color!

Still the human eye is only the outward projection of an intricate visual apparatus—consisting of the two eyes, the two optic nerves and, most important of all, the visual brain areas where images are received, interpreted and visual impressions stored.

The demands of civilization, in its increasing complexity, indirectly created impediments in all three parts of this visual apparatus: errors of refraction interfering with the optical focusing of the eyes, muscular irregularities inside and outside the eyes, pathological involvements affecting all parts, and mental abnormalities.

Optically, the refractive elements of the eye—the cornea and the lens, were efficient enough to focus correctly for distant objects. Early man could survive the many dangers, could prepare for fight or flight, could sight game or study the stars for guidance on land or sea. Natural selection eliminated those whose overall refraction was too poor for survival.

During early civilization, as farmer, hunter, trapper or seaman, man used his eyes almost exclusively for long-range, daylight seeing, just as nature intended. More and more, as close-seeing demands increased at an accelerating pace, the optical system of the eye lagged behind. Industrial and cultural develop-

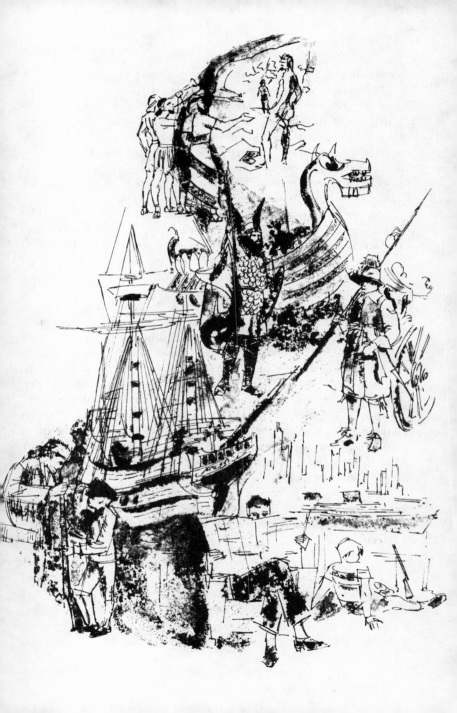

ments and their visual requirements found the eye, from an evolutionary point of view, quite unprepared.

Even distance-seeing demands in the world of modern civilization—with high speed transportation, nocturnal abuse of the eyes, increased artificial light stimulants such as television, movies, photographic and scientific instrument use, etc., became more exacting. Speed and accuracy in focusing, in perception, in muscle reaction, are required far in excess of nature's capability at the present stage of the eye's evolution.

Hence, it is not surprising that modern-day eyes rebel. The front corneal curve provided by nature as the prime refracting surface is simply not sufficiently accurate to properly refract to the fine focuses needed. Symptoms result because of this inability: headaches, blurred vision, double-vision, drowsiness, irritability, eye fatigue and pain.

Though the present-day eye has not changed materially from the day of the cave man, it is clear that the tasks it must face have changed radically. We could no doubt use our eyes as well as the ancient cave man—if they were used for the same purpose. Nor would we have visual defects if this were the case. Basically, because our eyes are much healthier than were those in prehistoric or historic times, we should have far less visual defects.

But it is precisely because uses have changed and the eyes have not, that visual defects have developed; thus many of us must draw on our excess nervous energy (which we call strain) and in other ways assist our unadapted eyes in order to perform today's visual tasks.

Centuries from now the human eye may have adapted to extant needs, but in the meantime we must employ artificial and externally applied remedies and devices in order to correct these defects.

III

What Troubles the Eye?

Everyone who has used a camera knows that to obtain a clear picture the camera must be in focus. The same principle applies to the eye. The image formed by the eye's optical system is identical with that formed by an ordinary lens or lens combination. As a matter of fact, if the back of an actual eye is removed a tiny image forms on paper held in its place.

Figures 12A and 12B show the normal eye perfectly in focus, with images of both distant and near objects falling squarely on the retina.

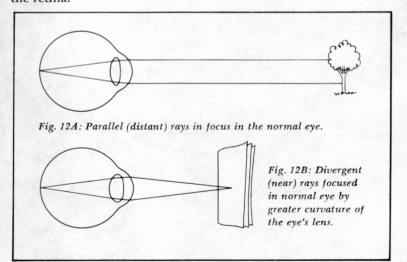

Fig. 12A: Parallel (distant) rays in focus in the normal eye.

Fig. 12B: Divergent (near) rays focused in normal eye by greater curvature of the eye's lens.

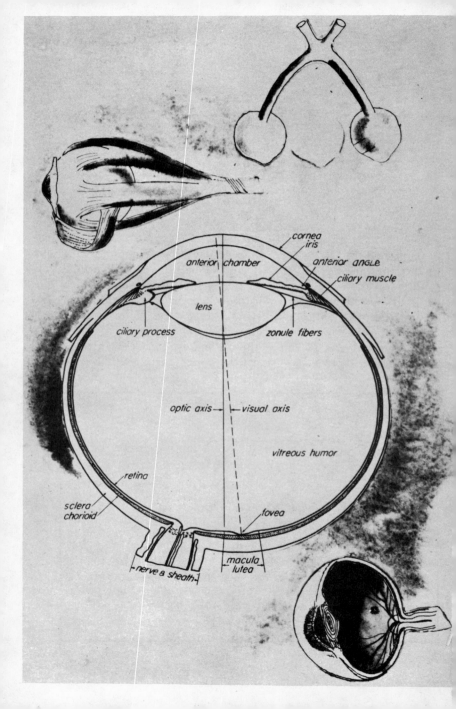

But frequently the image of a distant object falls in front of the retina. This is because of excessive focusing power in relation to the eye's dimensions (front to rear) —more than 80% of this focusing power due to the cornea and less than 20% due to the crystalline lens. The image is therefore out of focus at the retina and unclear.

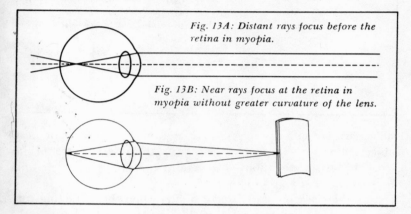

Fig. 13A: Distant rays focus before the retina in myopia.

Fig. 13B: Near rays focus at the retina in myopia without greater curvature of the lens.

Figure 13A depicts myopia, commonly called nearsightedness. All objects beyond 20 feet are focused as shown here. Only objects relatively close to the individual (within 20 ft.) are focused clearly on the retina (Fig. 13B)

On the other hand, an image, because of inadequate focusing by the cornea and the lens with relation to the length of the eye, may sometimes fall behind the retina. This does not mean an actual image is formed here (since the back layers of the eye are not transparent), but it does mean that the retina intercepts and is activated by rays of light which have not yet come to a focus. The image here, too, is out of focus and unclear.

Figures 14A and 14B demonstrate hyperopia, generally called far-sightedness. Objects beyond 20 feet are usually seen more clearly than those at a shorter distance, though they too are blurred. But this blur is masked because of the reserve focusing power in the crystalline lens which can be brought into play. When this is added to the corneal refracting power it is frequently

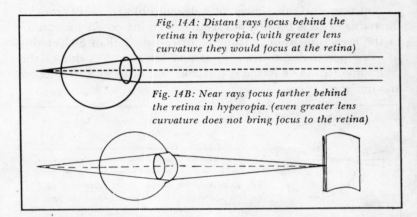

Fig. 14A: Distant rays focus behind the retina in hyperopia. (with greater lens curvature they would focus at the retina)

Fig. 14B: Near rays focus farther behind the retina in hyperopia. (even greater lens curvature does not bring focus to the retina)

sufficient, particularly in youth, to eliminate the blur. For near objects, however, especially in later years, this reserve power of the lens—the accommodation—is generally not strong enough and they consequently appear blurred.

Another lack of retinal focus occurs when the refracting surfaces, either cornea or crystalline lens or both, are not perfectly round. In such a case, for instance, rays of light in a vertical plane are not focused to the same extent as rays of light in a horizontal plane. This unequal focusing is called astigmatism, literally lack of a point, referring to the blurred focus.

Figure 15 shows this condition. Here, however, there is no difference in clarity between images from distant or near objects. Both are blurred.

These three are the most common refractive defects of the

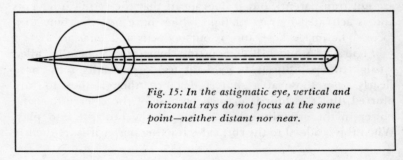

Fig. 15: In the astigmatic eye, vertical and horizontal rays do not focus at the same point—neither distant nor near.

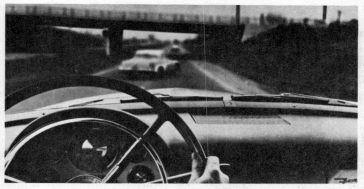

Fig. 16: In myopia note the blur at distance, the clarity at near.

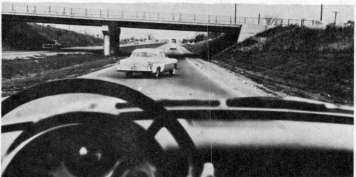

Fig. 17: In hyperopia note the blur at near, the clarity at distance.

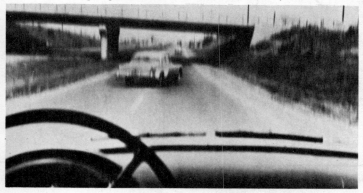

Fig. 18: In astigmatism note the blur at distance and near.
Photographs courtesy American Optical Co.

eye and are obviously due to improper focusing mechanisms—resulting in a refracting power inexactly related to the length of the eye. Primarily, the curvature of the front corneal surface is the culprit.

How these defects affect the visual impression formed by the images is readily apparent to anyone who has ever looked through someone else's glasses.

Abnormality of lens focusing is an inevitable byproduct of age. This condition is known as presbyopia, or old-sight, and results from the inability of the crystalline lens to focus on objects close at hand. Theories have this inability developing as a natural consequence of hardening of the lens tissues or as a weakening of the muscles controlling lens focusing. Whatever the reasons no one is immune, and it is a process which thus far has defied retardation.

Figure 19 shows the normal accommodating eye, with full ease of change of focus. Notice the greater roundness of the lens. Fig. 19A is of the presbyopic eye, which finds accommodation difficult or impossible.

It is fair to state that these four eye defects, separately and

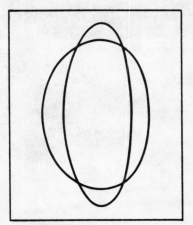

Fig. 19: The normal eye at near: lens rapidly assumes greater curvature.

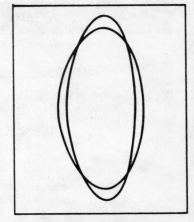

Fig. 19A: The presbyopic eye at near: lens tends to stay flat.

together, in differing degree and variation, account for 75 to 85% of all visual difficulties.

Of course, there are many other conditions leading directly and indirectly to refractive ills. Among these are muscular defects, cross-eyes, double vision, unequal image sizes between the two eyes, and others. But these are comparatively uncommon.

Infrequent too are the pathological involvements such as cataract, glaucoma, retinitis, neuritis, brain disorders, and a host of other diseases which may prey upon or leave their effect upon the visual apparatus.

But it is unquestioned that most ocular discomforts—headaches, eyeaches, irritability, inability to concentrate on a visual task, photophobia (aversion to light), and frequent eye fatigue—most commonly point to some focusing difficulty, some "error of refraction" linked to one of the four basic defects we have discussed.

In the case of near-sightedness there is always an unmistakable blur, because no mechanism within the eye can clear the focus.

In the case of farsightedness there is such a mechanism, and young people are often unaware of hyperopia because of their ability to utilize reserve refracting power of the lens to clarify the focus. The strain in utilizing this reserve power, however, causes the related symptoms—symptoms which the nearsighted individual does not experience.

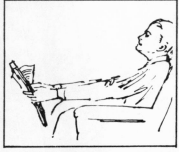

Fig. 20: Beginning signs of presbyopia: print must be moved further away.

Similarly, astigmatism produces strain and discomfort, although lens effort will sometimes partially compensate for the defect.

In its early stages, when it still can be overcome by excessive accommodative effort, presbyopia likewise produces headaches and related symptoms. Later on the focusing effort will be of no avail and is abandoned. When this happens only the blur is evident. Moving reading matter farther away clears the fuzziness, but only for a short time.

These, then, are the causes and effects of most defects which plague the human eye today.

Unmistakably, they all have a common source—the refractive inadequacy of the front corneal surface, with only presbyopia accentuating the role of the eye's crystalline lens.

IV

First Steps in Eye Correction

It is not always true that all eye defects necessarily need correcting. Eyes have always had some defects—from caveman days to the present. For example, investigations among people of different ages, classes and races indicate that a degree of hyperopia is practically normal and is associated with the keenest sight. Theoretically, this can be compared with the fine adjustments of a microscope. Everyone who has used a microscope knows an object can be seen in greater detail when the fine adjustment dial is manipulated to and fro, rather than when the focus is fixed. In nature, apparently, the ciliary muscle, which controls the focusing of the crystalline lens, similarly allows this slight play to and fro.

Moreover, cases have been recorded, even in recent years, of individuals who could see three of the planet Jupiter's moons with the naked eye. This requires an acuity (resolving power) at least four times that of the normal eye!

On the other hand, there have no doubt been millions of people who have gone through life without seeing clearly beyond ten or twenty feet. They could never clearly see the moon, the stars or a distant landscape, and never realized it.

A fair degree of astigmatism, too, is considered quite normal and generally overlooked.

Only when one of these conditions leads to a noticeable blurring or other symptoms of discomfort is relief sought.

So it must have been in the days of the caveman when, by

41

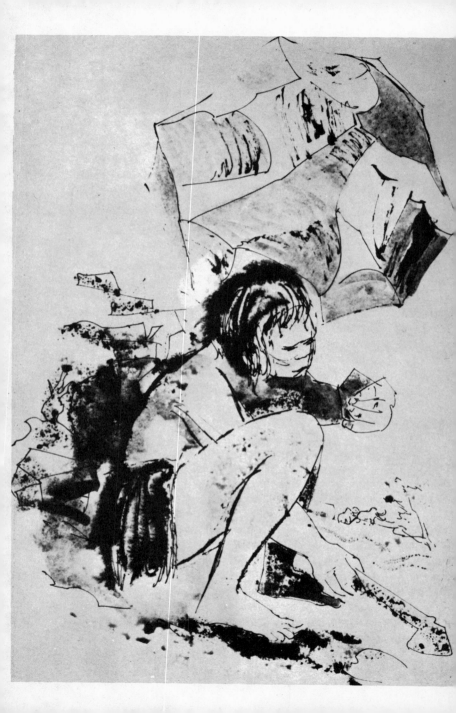

chance, he found that distant objects could be seen more clearly through a fragment of volcanic rock. This was a quartz or silicon crystal—a molten mass of silica sand, soda ash and lime which, upon cooling, assumed a molecular structure which permitted light to pass through.

Perhaps the caveman found that near objects seemed enlarged if viewed through a transparent fragment shaped a little differently than this rock which gave clearer distant vision. Possibly he rubbed these objects with moss, or hide, or sand, and found a high polish could be produced. This made objects look even clearer and produced reflections, too.

From these haphazard efforts came the birth of the lens and the mirror.

From this makeshift production of glass to the modern, man-made kind would appear to be just a simple step . . . but it must have been centuries before it was taken.

The Bible abounds with references to glass and glass manufacture. Jewelry designing and gem cutting as fine arts were practiced in Egypt as early as 500 B.C. Glass artifacts have been found in Egyptian tombs, and Minoan examples of lenses worked from rock crystals dating from 2000 to 1000 B.C. can be found in museums. The achievement of detail in this delicate work could hardly have been executed without the use of some visual aids.

The ancient Greeks assigned the origin of glass production to the accidental discovery by Phoenician merchants of a glasslike substance formed by the heat of their cooking pots on impure sodium carbonate and sand. In the ruins of Carthage, Greece's greatest colony, have been found magnifying lenses, and in the remains of Nineveh and Troy lenses have been discovered.

Yet it is an extraordinary thing that the Greeks, with their lively and penetrating minds, never realized the possibilities of either the microscope or the telescope—nor even the use of glass as an aid to vision. They made no acknowledged use of the lens. Still, they lived in a world where glass had been known and made beautiful for hundreds of years, and they had about them glass flasks and bottles through which they unquestionably must have caught glimpses of objects distorted and enlarged. But science in Greece was pursued by philosophers in an aristocratic spirit. These were men who, with few exceptions, like Archimedes, were too proud to learn from mere artisans such as jewelers and glass-workers.

Long before Roman times glass was used for the production of vases, mirrors and gems of all kinds. Euclid's works on optics, Plato's "Theory of Vision," Aristotle's familiarity with myopia and Archimedes fabled use of burning mirrors to destroy the Roman fleet are known to any student of antiquity.

In 50 B.C., Seneca, the Roman, produced references to convex lenses and prismatic colors caused by angular reflection. Ptolemy, in the second century after the birth of Christ, included studies of vision and the refraction of light in his thirteen philosophical volumes.

So it is not surprising to read that the Emperor Nero supposedly watched gladiatorial contests through an emerald or that the Romans believed nearsightedness diminished the value of a slave. Although records reveal that a glass bowl filled with water produced a magnifying effect (in effect a convex lens), the Romans apparently did not apply this to overcome presbyopia. Instead they allowed a slave to read to them. But this water lens was used by physicians to concentrate light and heat for healing purposes, so its focusing value did not entirely escape the Romans.

Even the writings of Confucius, in the China of 500 B.C., refer to the use of crystals to restore vision to a poor cobbler. Travelers' tales have made China the original center of glasses as we know them. Actually, the earliest evidence concerning glasses in China reveals they were discovered and used considerably later than the time they made their appearance in Europe. The use of crystals and gems as visual aids by Chinese, however, precedes their use in Europe. Repeated references and even illustrations of near-sighted mandarins using "concave" lenses to help them see distant objects are frequently found in medieval Chinese writings.

The ancient Roman and Greek belief that light emanated from the eye to produce vision—rather than originating from

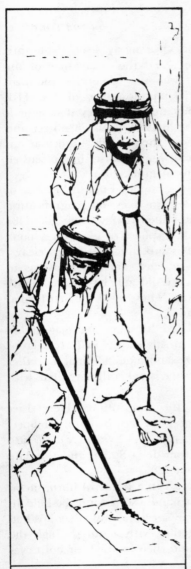

Fig. 22: Alhazen—965-1038 A.D.
—studied the refraction of
light and disputed the ancient
theory that visual rays
emanated from the eye.
(Bausch & Lomb)

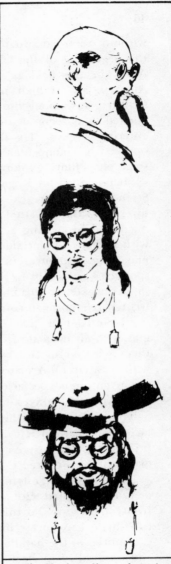

Fig. 23: According to legend
spectacles were born in the
time of Confucius—500 B.C.
Marco Polo reported them in
general use in China about
1275 A.D. (Bausch & Lomb)

without, retarded progress in optics for many years. Not until the beginning of the Christian era and the ascendancy of the Arabs in the field of learning, was this theory abandoned. Alhazen, an Arabian mathematician-philosopher of the 11th Century, was among the first to advance the theory that sight is elicited by a "cone of light rays emanating from an object and entering the eye." He also advanced theories of "binocular" as opposed to "monocular" vision, and for the first time discussed some elementary explorations into magnification.

It remained for Roger Bacon, the famous English "Father of Science," however, to apply the principles of magnification directly to the eye. In 1266 he explained that writing could be magnified by placing a segment of a sphere of glass on a book with its flat or plane side down. His subsequent writings clearly make him a pioneer in this new science, and his allusions to spectacles as "useful to those who are old and have weak sight" show the extent of his understanding. These were the first formal written references to corrective lenses.

Records show that Bacon related his ideas on magnifying glasses to an intimate friend, who in his travels in Italy relayed them to a Dominican friar, one Allessandro della Spina. Together with a Salvino d'Armato, della Spina is generally credited with the invention of spectacles.

D'Armato's gravestone bears the inscription "Here Lies Salvino d'Armato of the Amati of Florence. Inventor of Spectacles. God Pardon Him His Sins. A.D. 1317." Evidently d'Armato utilized the knowledge acquired from della Spina, and the date of invention is conceded to be about 1285.

At first the magnifying lens was set in a frame of horn, metal or wood, mounted with a short flat handle so it could be held in front of the eye. To this the name spectacle was given. When two single lenses were hinged together with a pin through the extremities of the handles, they could then be used for both eyes and were called spectacles.

Fleeting references to glasses and spectacles appear in medieval literature. Chaucer refers to them in his "The Wife's Tale" in 1386. So does a writer named Hoccleve in a manuscript of

1415. A fourteenth century writing in the Paris Bibliotheque Nationale pictures St. Paul holding spectacles. Francisco Redi, writing in 1676, refers to an old manuscript dated 1299 which says "without glasses known as spectacles, I have strength neither to read nor write. These have lately been invented for the convenience of poor old people who are weak-sighted."

But for many years the correction of visual defects other than presbyopia remained dormant. No advancement beyond Bacon's original concept was made. The stagnation in most scientific fields during this era also pervaded optics. Without question this stagnation could be ascribed to the fact that the Middle Ages was essentially a religious era and the Church was all-powerful. Its strength lay in man's preoccupation with heaven rather than with earth, and any scientific study was viewed as having little importance.

Also, both the clergy and the medical profession united in trying to suppress the doctoring of eyes with glasses as deliberate interference with God's purpose of afflicting the aged. Small wonder that progress was slow.

Four hundred years elapsed between Bacon's basic concept of eye correction and Dutchman Willebrord Snell's elementary law of refraction. This simple law explained in mathematical terms the principles of optics utilized in lenses, telescopes, micro-

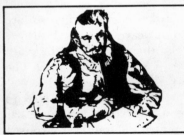

Fig. 24A: Willebrord Snell discovered the law of refraction in 1621. This law makes possible precise computation of modern lenses and optical instruments. (Bausch & Lomb)

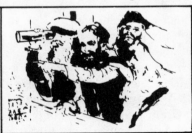

Fig. 24B: In 1609 Galileo was acclaimed by distinguished citizens of Venice when he demonstrated his first telescope from the tower of St. Marks. (Bausch & Lomb)

scopes, indeed in all optical instruments. In 1621 he expressed this as his sine law, discovering that when light falls upon the surface of a transparent medium—such as glass or water, the angle which it makes with the surface bears a constant ratio to the angle it assumes in the new medium.

Galileo's demonstration of the first telescope, Huygens' wave theory of light, Descartes' optical writings, "La Dioptrique," Newton's "Optiks," were all contemporary to Snell and indicated the great awakening of interest in the field of optics.

Unwittingly making use of Snell's law, the guiding concept of eye correction had been to provide external refractive means either to add to or subtract from the under- or over-refraction of the eye's optical system. To this day the science of eye correction is based on this.

Reduced to essentials this theory utilized the light-bending properties of a curved transparent surface. It was found that when light hit a surface obliquely (or struck a curved surface) its rays were either brought together (converged) or separated (diverged). This depended, as Snell discovered, first on the so-called refractive index of the new medium entered (the rate at which light travels in this medium), and second on the thickness of the medium.

A prism is a fundamental example of such a medium. As Fig. 25A shows, it is a three-surfaced piece of glass of unequal dimension. When a ray of light strikes the entering surface obliquely (at an angle), or when it leaves the final surface obliquely, it is then bent toward the thicker part of the glass. This is because the speed of light is lessened by the glass. The thicker the glass the more are the rays of light retarded.

Applying this principle of a prism, it is a simple step to envision joining two prisms together at the bases or thicker parts to produce convergence toward the center. Substantially a convex lens results. Joining two prisms at the apices or thinner parts gives divergence toward the edges—the effect of a "concave" lens. Basically, therefore, the light principle involved is identical both for prisms and lenses (Fig. 25B).

Sir Isaac Newton was the first to discover that a prism dis-

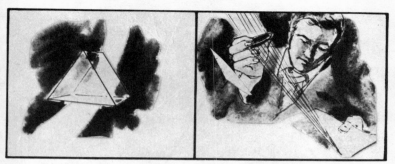

Fig. 25A: Light refraction
through a prism. Note oblique
incidence.

Fig. 25B: Light refraction
through a curved surface.

persed white light into various colors (a rainbow effect). He
determined that the "primary" colors were red, green, and blue,
and combinations of these produced all the others. James C.
Maxwell (1873) devised an ingenious color triangle which later
proved useful in showing how all colors combined. (Fig. 25C
and 25D.)

Figure 26A shows the effect of parallel rays of light on a
convex or magnifying lens—used to counteract hyperopia and to

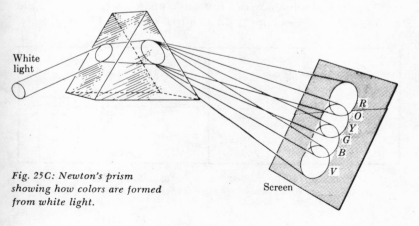

White
light

R
O
Y
G
B
V

Screen

Fig. 25C: Newton's prism
showing how colors are formed
from white light.

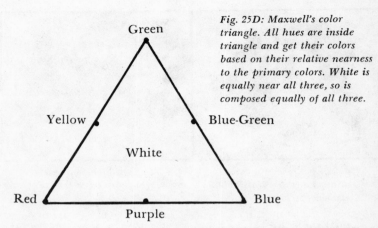

Green

Yellow   Blue-Green

White

Red   Blue

Purple

Fig. 25D: Maxwell's color triangle. All hues are inside triangle and get their colors based on their relative nearness to the primary colors. White is equally near all three, so is composed equally of all three.

add to deficient refraction. Fig. 26B shows the effect of a concave or minifying lens—used to counteract myopia and, by diverging the rays, to detract from an over-refraction.

The first simple, single focus bi-convex and bi-concave lenses shown here were used for many centuries—and there were no lenses at all for astigmatic conditions until the nineteenth century, when this condition was identified. Until then the convex lens was used for hyperopia and presbyopia, and the concave lens for myopia.

The first graphic portrayal of any apparatus utilizing simple forms of these lenses appears in a church fresco at Trevisco, Italy.

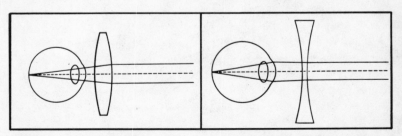

Fig. Fig. 26A: Parallel light rays being converged by a convex lens.

Fig. 26B: Parallel light rays being diverged by a concave lens.

Painted in 1352, it shows a Cardinal Ugone wearing two mounted lenses with their handles riveted together and fixed in front of his eyes. But the first medical reference to glasses—and that somewhat deprecatory—was by a professor at Montpelier in 1305 who recommended an eye salve of such potency that "it will enable those whose sight is weak . . . to read without glasses."

A painting by Raphael in 1517 depicted Pope Leo X as holding a concave glass—the first known use of such a lens in Western civilization. But it is generally accepted that convex lenses came into common use in the mid-fourteenth century.

In addition to religious objections to glasses, very few people of this era were literate, so the demand for visual correction, particularly for close-range work, could not have been pronounced. Real impetus came later on, in the fifteenth century, when the invention of movable type and the circulation of the printed word focused attention on the difficulties of reading vision. Thereafter, the demand for convex lenses as an aid to reading grew rapidly and the trade in spectacles mushroomed, especially in North Italy and Germany where glassworkers were predominant.

By 1600 literacy was increasing, religious influence was on the wane, scientific interest in optics had blossomed, and a new trade was recognized: opticians were to be found in most towns of any size in Europe.

Something akin to mass production of glasses evolved in England late in the seventeenth century with the introduction of lens grinding in large numbers on one large block. This development gave London spectacle manufacturers a substantial advantage over their foreign rivals from the standpoint of both price and quality. Records indicate that the best double-jointed gold-rimmed spectacles, with gold case included, commanded a price of sixteen guineas ($80). At this time these manufacturers also introduced the monocle, or single eye lens, identified to this day with the English nobleman.

Bifocal lenses—those ground with one portion for distant focusing and the other for near—came on the scene in 1784, a manifestation of the genius of Benjamin Franklin.

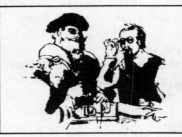 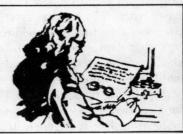

Fig. 27A: In Europe from the
14th to 17th centuries, street
vendors sold crude spectacles,
both for adornment and as
an aid to vision. (Bausch &
Lomb)

Fig. 27B: Benjamin Franklin
by his invention of the bifocal
lens in 1784 gave the great
gift of youthful vision to
generation of spectacle wearers.

For a long time spectacles or eyeglasses, as they came to be called, were not well received by oculists—physicians specializing in eye care. Even after the highly esteemed German astronomer Johannes Kepler did considerable theoretical work in optics, giving it the stamp of orthodoxy, the use of drugs rather than lenses in cases of weak sight was preferred. Oculists could not conceive how an "eye that does not see well would see better with something in front of it."

Nevertheless, treatises published by humble vendors of glasses systematized a great deal of practical and useful information concerning their use. In 1623 one such publication appeared in Seville, Spain, clearly indicating the use of "high convex lenses after cataract operation" and laid down a scale of .different strength of reading glasses for different ages.

Almost down to the middle of the nineteenth century, the fitting of glasses was the prerogative of untrained vendors, mostly itinerant, who combined this business with other occupations identified with peddlers. Oculists took but the slightest interest in glasses, at best recommending a patient visit a shop and select the most suitable pair.

The range of choice, of course, was not wide. The stock in trade consisted of glasses for use after cataract operation, glasses

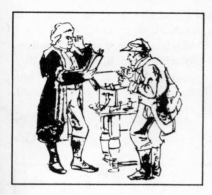

Fig. 27C: "The Eyglass Vendor." Painted in 1864. (Bausch & Lomb)

for old sight, glasses for short sight, and occasionally glasses for "old sight of young people"—a phrase denoting farsightedness.

Astigmatism was not known until 1801 when Thomas Young made a demonstration of it with his own eyes and published his chief work, "The Mechanism of the Eye." That a corrective lens for this defect was possible was not realized until the English physicist Airy devised a suitable cylindrical lens in 1827. However, not until after Donders had anticipated, about 1850, the modern tool of retinoscopy (a means of tracing a ray of light onto the human retina), was correction of astigmatism practical.

Also in the 1850s the so-called Snellen chart for distance testing was introduced by an English oculist. It provided a means for comparing visual acuity with an accepted norm, and in its modern form enables the eye examiner to evaluate vision as a fraction: 20/20 signifying that the individual can see at 20 feet what the normal eye sees at 20 feet; 20/40 signifying that the individual can see at 20 feet what the normal eye sees at 40 feet, etc.

Likewise, the Jaeger test types for near visual acuity were applied in similar fashion by Snellen. The use of the term diopter as a unit of lens measure was not adopted until 1875; previously, the English inch system was used. The diopter refers to a unit of focal power of one meter (39.37 inches) and is universally in use today.

The introduction by Helmholtz, the German physiologist, in the 1850s of the ophthalmoscope—the instrument designed for viewing the internal portion of the eye, and the work of Donders, von Graefe and countless other physicians and physiologists during the mid-nineteenth century, made problems of refraction and use of corrective glasses acceptable as part of the eye physician's creed.

The use of prisms, per se, also dates from this period. Fig. 28 shows how a prism changes the direction of a ray of light. This

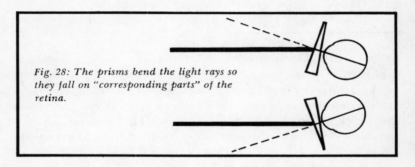

Fig. 28: The prisms bend the light rays so they fall on "corresponding parts" of the retina.

property is useful in cases of turned or crossed eyes in order to permit the focusing of like images on the same parts of the retinas in both eyes. Single vision with both eyes then is favored. The use of prisms in this conection and in cases of muscular insufficiency—where an eye may have only a weakness or tendency to turn, stems from the work of Kepler and Wells in 1792. The clinical work of Donders in 1847 and of von Graefe in 1857 added much to this study.

Countless more names might be mentioned. The history of optics is replete with names like da Vinci, Leeuwenhoek, Fraunhofer. All contributed heavily to the vast sum of knowledge accumulated in the field of optics. But through it all—from the day original glasses were worn by Cardinal Ugone to the present— the simple concept of utilizing a concave lens for near-sightedness, a convex lens for far-sightedness and presbyopia, and a cylindrical lens for astigmatism has been retained, all in the form of one or two pieces of glass supported by a frame resting on the nose.

Spectacle frames have a history of their own, too. They ran the gamut from metal to leather. Glasses were secured by a tape tucked under the hat (a method reminiscent of the Chinese way of binding glasses to headgear). Various forms of lorgnettes—from ear-rails to stringed nosepieces, have had their day.

Gold, silver, steel, fish-bone, horn, wood, ivory and leather have all been employed in the making of spectacle frames. Plastic is the most modern substance used to support glasses.

Basically, though, frames have remained unchanged through the years. They remain a simple device to hold two pieces of glass in front of the eyes.

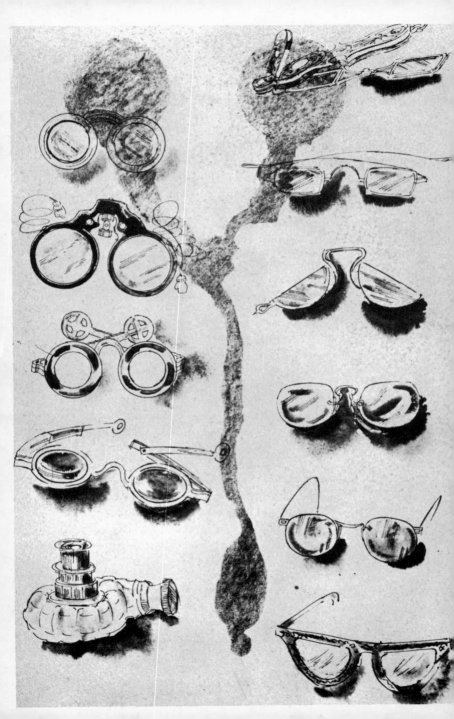

V
Glasses Become Commonplace

With glasses coming of age as an accepted form of therapy for eye defects, new methods of eye testing evolved.

The ophthalmoscope, in addition to bringing forward a wealth of new clinical concepts in pathology—retinitis pigmentosa, glioma of the retina, sarcoma of the choroid, retinal detachment, and retinal and vitreous disease processes due to bodily disorders—also served to open the door to objective determination of refractive errors.

The application of its fundamental principle—casting a concentrated beam of light into the eye, and its methods—a point source of light reflected to enable an observer through a centered opening to view the light directly along its path, resulted in probably the greatest objective aid of all—the retinoscope—invented in 1871 by a French oculist, Cuignet.

Helmholtz's work on the ophthalmoscope (along with contributions by Jaeger) led him to devise the instrument known today the ophthalmometer—utilizing principles of reflection to measure the curvature of the corneal surface. An original instrument of this nature built by Javal in 1872 still serves as the model of modern instruments.

More and more, as these instruments, lenses and others came into use, the fitting of glasses ceased to be a matter of trial and error and became what we know today as the science of Optometry, literally eye-measurement.

As recently as fifty years ago, selecting corrective lenses was

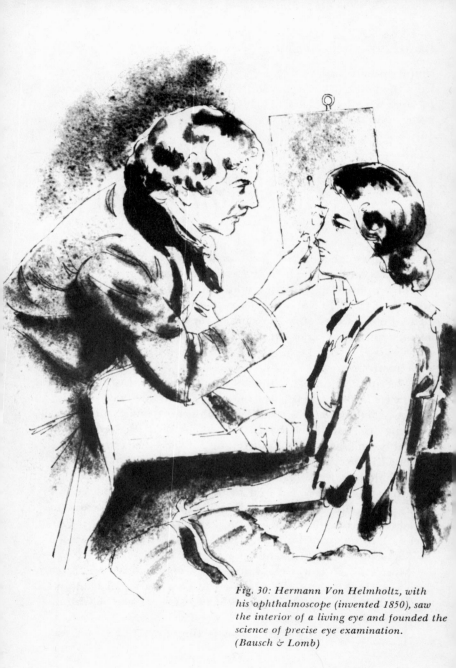

Fig. 30: Hermann Von Helmholtz, with
his ophthalmoscope (invented 1850), saw
the interior of a living eye and founded the
science of precise eye examination.
(Bausch & Lomb)

simply a matter of buying a pair of glasses, hardly an advance from the ignorance of the Middle Ages. The steps a person went through to get glasses are well illustrated by Benjamin Franklin's letter to his sister in July, 1771 (though we could easily substitute July, 1910).

"Dear Sister,

I thought you had mentioned in one of your letters a desire to have spectacles of some sort sent you, but I cannot now find such a letter. However, I send you a pair of every size of glasses from 1 to 13. To suit yourself, take a pair at a time, and hold one of the glasses first against one eye and then against the other, looking at some small print.

If the first suits neither eye, put them up again before you open a second. Thus you will keep them from mixing.

By trying and comparing at your leisure, you may find those that are best for you, which you cannot do well in a shop, where for want of time and care, people often take such as strain their eyes and hurt them.

I advise you trying each of your eyes separately, because few people's eyes are fellows, and almost everybody in reading or working uses one eye principally, the other being dimmer or perhaps fitter for distant objects, and thence it happens that the spectacles, whose glasses are fellows suit sometimes that eye which before was not used, though they do not suit the other.

When you have suited yourself, keep the higher numbers for future use as your eyes may grow older, and oblige your friends with the others.

With best wishes for you, and yours, I am ever

Yours affectionate brother
B. Franklin"

Many older persons may still recall people going to the "five and ten" or department stores to get a new pair of spectacles because the old ones had worn out. Indeed, in many countries outside the United States this is still the practice, and there is no restriction or regulation on prescribing or fitting glasses.

Nevertheless, the vast accomplishments of Donders, the Dutch physician regarded as the father of modern refraction, added to those of Helmholtz, Tscherning, Fresnel, Gauss, Maxwell, Tyndall and other English physicists, have borne luxurious fruit. And the science of refraction today has taken its place on a par wtih other medical ancillary callings such as Dentistry.

How are glasses fitted?

In general, modern methods include the use of both subjective and objective means.

Anyone who has had his eyes tested for glasses recalls that after describing his symptoms or complaints, he was asked to read a chart from a distance of anywhere from 10 to 20 feet. This is the first step in a procedure called the subjective findings.

The Snellen chart used here has already been discussed. It is a chart consisting of square-shaped letters arranged in diminishing size. The height of each letter subtends an angle of five minutes (1/12 of a degree) if viewed at certain distances. The large

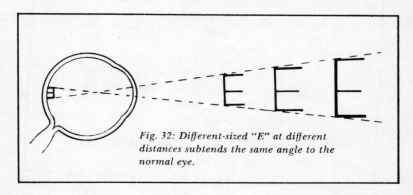

Fig. 32: Different-sized "E" at different distances subtends the same angle to the normal eye.

E, for instance, subtends this angle at 200 feet, the next smaller letters at 100 feet, then at 70, 50, 40, 30, 20, 15 and 10 feet. Fig. 32 shows this in relation to the eye.

In this manner, if the large letter E cannot be seen at 200 feet but only at 20 feet, vision is expressed as 20/200. If your sight is normal you will see the letter at 20 feet which subtends an angle of five minutes or which the normal eye sees at 20 feet. Your vision is 20/20. Many persons, especially during youth, can read the line which should be read at 15 or even 10 feet when they are 20 feet away. The fractions here would be 20/15 or 20/10.

The Snellen fraction does not represent the fraction of normal vision; it is merely a recording device. 20/40, for instance, does not mean 50% vision, any more than 20/200 means 10% vision. The fraction is simply a convenient way to record the relative ability to read at 20 feet letters which normally are seen at other distances. It is a guide to the extent of visual impairment.

Other charts are commonly used for illiterates or children. In many eye-tests letters are projected on a screen and the chart is not used. Its purpose is nevertheless the same. Substantially, this reading of a chart with the eyes separately and together commonly introduces the subjective phase.

A near chart is employed to test the focusing power of the crystalline lens—the eye's internal lens. This is the so-called Jaeger test-types—simply a number of paragraphs of different-sized letters ranging from approximately half typewriter print to about double. Each paragraph is numbered and the smallest letters viewed are known as J1, J2, etc. This is a guide, also, to the extent of accommodative impairment—especially significant, as we have mentioned, in presbyopia.

At this point in the eye-test the "objective" phase usually intervenes. The ophthalmoscope is used to view the surfaces of the eye, the media (the anterior chamber, lens, posterior chamber), and the back of the eye—the retina or fundus. This reveals any pathological condition or any deviation from normal, and also provides valuable clues (because of the lens power needed in the ophthalmoscope to produce clear vision) as to the refrac-

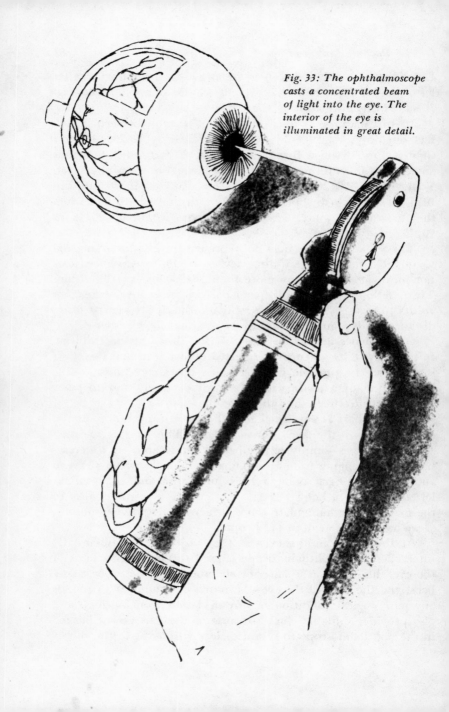

Fig. 33: The ophthalmoscope casts a concentrated beam of light into the eye. The interior of the eye is illuminated in great detail.

tive state of the eye. Here, you will recall, you have been directed to look at a distant point while the viewer approaches your eye very closely with a concentrated beam of light from a small hand instrument.

When you place your head on a rather imposing instrument and your chin upon a specially designed rest, your eyes are being checked with the ophthalmometer we spoke of earlier (also called the keratometer). Through a small tube you will see the observer's eye and he, in turn, will view your eye and will align several images depending upon the curvature of the cornea. In this way, the cornea—be it spherical, astigmatic, or irregular, can be measured.

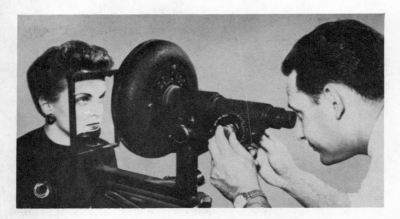

Fig. 34: The ophthalmometer measures the precise curvature of the cornea's central surface. It is invaluable for astigmatism.

A trial frame—exactly what the name states, is now placed before the eyes. Trial lenses are placed in this frame to determine their suitability to your eyes. Today all trial lenses are inserted simultaneously into one large instrument—the phoropter, and can be rotated into position in front of the eyes.

Usually, heavy convex lenses are then placed in the phoropter or trial frame and you are directed to view a letter on the chart or a light on the screen. The purpose of the heavy convex lens

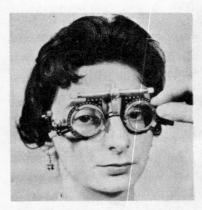

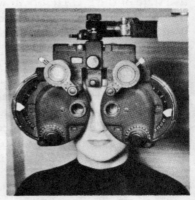

Fig. 35A: Trial lenses are inserted in the trial frame to test vision and muscular reactions.

Fig. 35B: The "phoropter" contains all the lenses necessary for eye-testing.

is to relax the accommodation of the eye, so it becomes inactive and does not affect the refraction of the eye when the distant letter is viewed (as it would in hyperopia). The letter, because of the lens, appears blurred—but this is expected.

Now the retinoscope is employed, casting parallel beams of light through the strong convex lens. Because of this lens, the light is refracted in a precise, expected way if your eye has no refractive error. This is readily seen when the light returns to the observer's eye. Any deviation of refraction can be measured, since other lenses can then be added in order to refract to the expected focus. Thus the total refraction of the eye can be ascertained in a simple yet very exact and wholly objective method. As a means of prescribing proper lens power without active cooperation from the person tested, the retinoscope is unsurpassed.

When the exact indication of your refractive condition is noted, the approximate correcting lens is placed in the phoropter. You are then asked to tell whether the letters on the chart are seen "better this way or that way?" while lenses—sometimes weaker, sometimes stronger, are added to this objective finding.

More often than not slight refinements are made which further improve visual acuity when the fine discrimination of the eye is called into play.

In the case of astigmatism where light rays in the vertical meridian may produce a sharper image than those in the horizontal meridian (or vice versa or obliquely, as the case may be) you are then asked, "which lines appear darker?" Proper cylindrical lenses—which clear up one meridian without affecting the other, are then applied to the point where all appear equally clear.

When each eye sees a different image, either above each other or side by side, a prism correction is applied until they fuse into a single image.

In this way you arrive at that combination of lenses—spherical and cylindrical, and prisms which produces the finest visual acuity and single binocular vision.

The eyes are tested both singly and binocularly to uncover not only the individual refractive error, but problems of association and dissociation of the two eyes, or muscular insufficiency or over-sufficiency. Corrective means, in the form of exercises or prisms, are then advised.

In brief, this is how you are tested for glasses—your refractive error is pinpointed, and, if your symptoms of eye discomfort are due to this effect, glasses to correct them are prescribed and fabricated. Two pieces of glass—precision-ground and flawlessly compounded, are then set in a frame or mounted with nose-piece and ear-pieces and are worn approximately one inch in front of your defective eyes. These are your new glasses.

Wherein are their limitations? In many and diverse respects.

Severe limitations have always been known and persist to this day. Quite apart from all factors relating to appearance and personality, conventional eyeglasses had and have certain well-recognized shortcomings with regard to visual utility.

For one, the field of corrected vision is necessarily limited by the dimensions of the refracting windows held in a fixed framework. In order to gain proper usage from glasses you must look *only* through the two panes of glass. When you look to the left or right, up or down, anywhere beyond the area of the glasses, they obviosuly lose their function.

From the field of vision of the normal uncorrected eye—which extends outward at least 90°, upward about 55°, downward approximately 70°, and inward close to 60°, there is a reduction of more than 25° in all directions. This becomes a serious handicap in many occupations.

Second, if your glasses are strong—if they exceed, to be generous, four or five diopters (generally linked to a visual acuity of 20/200 uncorrected or worse) —you can gain maximum visual benefit if you look only through the exact center of the lens. Looking through its peripheral area produces what scientists call marginal or spherical aberration, recognized commonly as blurring. This aberration is directly variable with the power of the lens. As a matter of fact, it is actually proportional to the cube of the power (3 x 3 x 3 with a 3 diopter lens, 2 x 2 x 2 with a 2 diopter lens) . Thus we have a 27x aberration in the first and an 8x aberration in the second. A person 3 diopters nearsighted sees objects peripherally blurred about three times as badly as one 2 diopters nearsighted, and as much as twenty-seven times as blurred as one only 1 diopter nearsighted or who needs no correction at all. Fortunately, this blurring is not too severe in mild corrections, but it is obvious how severe it may become in really strong ones.

Moreover, with strong lenses so-called induced astigmatism occurs as the result of oblique viewing. In addition, the effect of looking through a prism is introduced, creating displacement of the apparent position of objects. Where the prescription of each lens differs, an unequal displacement and frequently double-vision results, since the objects do not appear in the same place in space. The stronger your prescription, obviously the more pronounced is this displacement and double vision.

Third, eyeglasses are perched some distance from the eye—approximately one inch. Rays of light, therefore, after being refracted by the glass must pass through another medium—air—before entering the eye. The slightest tilting of the glasses (more so in strong prescriptions), has a disturbing effect. It means also that light rays falling upon the glasses from the rear—such as from a light behind the shoulder, can create disturbing reflections.

Fourth, there is an actual change in the size of images because of the distance between the glasses and the eyes. The combination of the focal system of the glass and the eye produces a new focal system resulting in a changed image size. For this reason a convex lens, quite apart from its refractive power, will make you see things larger than they actually are. If you are farsighted, therefore, you will get faulty perception and remote objects will appear larger and nearer.

A concave lens makes things appear smaller. Consequently, if you are nearsighted, objects will seem smaller and more distant. (A vicious cycle is created here, making the nearsighted person even more withdrawn and apart from his surroundings.)

This image-size difference becomes quite a problem, not so much when both eyes are equally near or farsighted, but when their refraction is unequal. One eye may be normal, the other nearsighted or farsighted; or the same defect may be present in different degrees.

Cases of aphakia present enormous difficulties. Here, one eye has undergone a cataract operation, and a very strong convex lens is required to compensate for the loss of the eye's crystalline lens. The good eye retains its original image size. However, to the eye subjected to surgery, objects viewed with the spectacle lens appear approximately 25% larger.

Small wonder that in many such cases one eye, usually the unaffected eye, must be prevented from seeing by occluding it with an opaque lens to avoid double vision. (Our discussion of oblique astigmatism and prismatic effect is likewise very much applicable here.)

Fifth, there are certain optical defects which simply cannot be corrected by conventional eyeglasses. Any ocular condition which gives an irregular shape to the cornea, and any lack of sphericity above a moderate amount of astigmatism, is virtually uncorrectable. This is because today's ophthalmic lenses can be ground only in spherical or cylindrical form, and therefore can correct only spherical or cylindrical discrepancies.

A classic example of this situation is keratoconus, where the cornea assumes a bulging, cone-like shape. Of unknown origin, this defect, or perhaps more properly called disease, is fortunately uncommon. Yet it occurs with sufficient frequency to cause it to be considered a serious problem.

It was first described in 1729 by the oculist Duddel who, in the case of a 14-year-old boy with the affliction, used substantially these words: "It is a change in the form of the cornea by which it takes the form of a cone, whose apex is blunt, but whose base is equal to the diameter of the cornea, which preserves its transparency." Another reference is made by a Dr. William Rowley (1743-1806) who spoke of it as follows: "A person formerly applied to me who had a convexity of the cornea, that formed a conic point like the top of a sugar loaf, which no glasses could remedy. This remarkable case happened from crying loud in hard labor."

The only reference to correcting keratoconus, prior to modern times, is made in the writings of the famous English architect Sir Christopher Wren, who attempted its correction with an unsuccessful hyperbolic lens in 1669. Because of the cornea's departure from a regular spherical or sphero-cylindrical surface, keratoconus as well as other corneal distortions such as scarring, has never been successfully corrected by ordinary glasses.

Sixth, there is a practical limit, weight-wise, to the strength to which regular glasses can be ground and still not be too heavy for certain strong prescriptions—despite the use of special glass of greater refractive index (thinlite). Further, serious practical difficulties arise in the actual grinding of unusually strong prescriptions.

Seventh, absolutely perfect alignment of frames, nosepiece, and earpiece must prevail in many prescriptions. Otherwise the optical axis of the lens will not coincide with that of the eye. Decentration effects and prismatic errors become evident. Discomfort, doubling and bothersome vision results.

And eighth, as many eyeglass wearers know to their dismay, ordinary glasses can be useless under conditions of rain, sleet, snow or fog. Entering a warm room from the cold outdoors can be an annoying experience. Certain occupations where passing in and out of a cold chamber is essential make glasses impractical. Firefighting, seafaring, fishing, certain types of flying and mining, as well as sports, all make eyeglass-wearing a problem.

Inevitably, as modern improvements in optometric and ophthalmologic testing technique developed and more exact visual analyses were possible, as new eye dysfunctions requiring precise correction were recognized and as lens production methods were perfected to the nth degree of quality standards, it became apparent that most of the above conditions of use posed virtually inescapable disadvantages to eyeglasses.

To some extent factors of marginal aberration and induced astigmatism were found conquerable. Modern astigmatically-corrected ophthalmic lenses such as Orthogon or Tillyer were introduced to make possible the diminution of the variation of strength between the center and the edge of the lens—the cause of the aberration.

The others, however, still remain and are handicaps still borne by today's beleaguered eyeglass wearer.

How do we eliminate them?

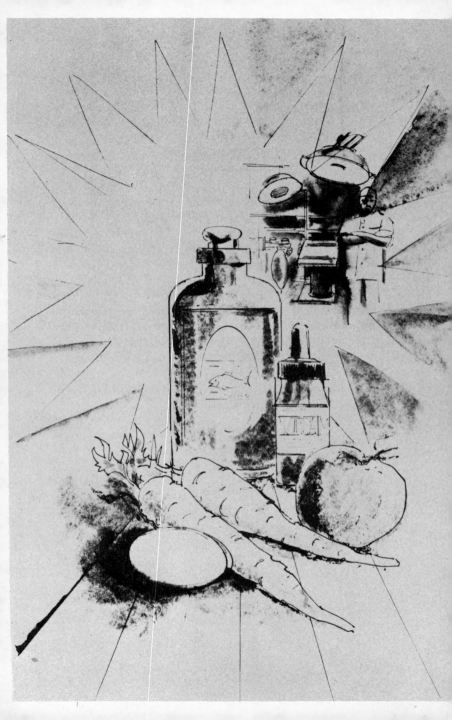

VI
Not with Glasses

Though we have traced the development of eyeglasses as the predominant form of sight correction, it should not be inferred that they were necessarily the only means of neutralizing or remedying eye defects.

We have noted that the eye physician and the oculist spurned the use of glasses for visual correction until well into the nineteenth century.

What remedy did he recommend before? And, for that matter, what remedies are utilized now?

History tells us that at one time the physician did little to actually remedy an eye defect. Resultant symptoms such as headaches, malaise, and eye-aches were treated as such with simple medication—the usual application directly to the eye taking the form of an eye salve.

Whether these symptoms were recognized as the result of refractive errors is not known. There were certainly no drugs specifically designed for refractive errors, although records show that in the thirteenth century one Ali ben Isa recommended that "they who do not see in the near, a condition which mainly affects old people, should use styptic medicines; whilst those who see well nearby but not in the distance, require medicines which give moist principle to the eye."

As late as the 1880s morphine, antipyrine, antifebrin and the like were commonly prescribed to relieve eyestrain. As soon as the therapeutic powers of lens correction were accepted and utilized, however, certain symptoms were relieved. Others did

not seem to be ameliorated. Research established that in some
cases the apparent need for lens correction was due to systemic
conditions.

Of late more and more refractive conditions—even myopia
(which produces little symptom of eyestrain), have been traced
to systemic origins and the proper dietary and medicinal means
employed to reduce or eliminate them.

Perhaps no condition more frequently leads to the conclusion
of eyestrain than headache. Most people will immediately blame
their headaches on their eyes. This is often justifiable since refractive errors and muscular defects will produce headache symptoms.
In these instances the pain is spoken of as dull or drawing—along
the brow and in or between the eyes. Movies, television, reading
or sewing may induce or aggravate headaches.

Headaches resulting from car-sickness or train-sickness are
due in some measure to eyestrain. Astigmatism and a muscular
defect generally predispose to this.

Glare or annoying reflections will sometimes produce headaches. This too should be eliminated with refractive corrections.
Other headaches may of course result from diseases of the eye,
such as glaucoma where there is a dull ache which may on
occasion be excruciating.

In general, those headaches which can be traced to ocular
origin can be fairly well localized. (Fig. 37.)

Certain other types of headaches—formerly ascribed to ocular

*Fig. 37: Frontal headaches
are commonly caused by
eye-strain.
Temporal headaches and those
at the back of the head
and neck are occasionally
caused by eyestrain and
generally by astigmatism,
muscular defect and excessive
glare.
Glaucoma, iritis, etc., cause
frontal pain and pain at the
back of the eye.*

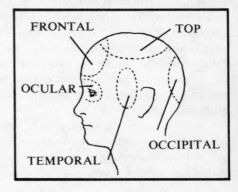

origin, have been found to be caused by neurosis or anemia in young people, and by high blood pressure among the middle- and old-aged. Intracranial lesions such as tumors may cause headaches at any age.

Giddiness—which may co-exist with a refractive error, is not infrequently traced to other causes. In older people it may be due to high blood pressure, in younger persons to a momentary insufficiency of blood supply to the brain.

Sinus conditions have been recognized as a chief cause of ocular, or apparent ocular, pains. Other toxic conditions throughout the body, in the teeth and the ears, for example, have been pinpointed as sources of ocular discomfort. Changes in the visual field, diplopia (double vision), and impairment of central vision are often treated as nerve disorders, quite independently of refractive errors. In many cases mitigation of the ocular symptoms results from specific nerve therapy.

Allergies will frequently cause ocular discomfort leading to the suspicion of refractive defect. Itching, tearing and photophobia linked frequently to conjunctivitis, are presumptive evidences of allergy, rather than need for refractive correction. Even keratitis and iritis (inflammations of the cornea and iris) result from this hyper-sensitivity.

Similarly, in the course of other systemic conditions—diseases such as diabetes (hyperglycemia, the oversupply of sugar) and its opposite (hypoglycemia, the under-supply of sugar), refractive conditions are created or masked which do not call for refractive correction. Occasionally there is an onset of myopia in the early stages of diabetes or during early treatment, increasing slowly and reaching high degrees within several months. This is because of changes within the crystalline lens which are more or less permanent. They may be the precursor of cataract. Diagnosis and therapy here is of the diabetes, and only secondarily of the myopia.

General mistiness, an inability to focus when reading (simulating presbyopia), and diplopia may seem to indicate a need for refractive aid, but the underlying cause may be hypoglycemia or an over-supply of insulin—hyperinsulinism.

Similarly, kidney ailments (nephritis) may change the index of refraction of the eye's media and thus affect its refraction. Syphilis is noted for its resemblance to many other afflictions, and it simulates refractive difficulties as well—particularly muscular and reflex defects.

Leukemia, in its advanced stage, produces night blindness as well as contraction of the fields of vision.

Pregnancy, because of its effect on the body glands, is known to produce refractive changes, and in extreme cases may cause toxemia (poisonous products in the blood). Although refraction may be severely affected by this condition, primary treatment is directed against the toxemia.

Aside from these general body conditions, there are specific eye affections which influence refraction and hence reveal themselves either as defective vision or strain.

Growths on the lid, such as a stye, may cause astigmatism by their pressure on the cornea. The failure of the lids to close properly may lead to astigmatism in some cases, myopia in others, by the effect on the corneal tissue.

Swellings, tumors or scars of the conjunctiva—the membrane lining the lid and the eye, may alter the mobility of the eye and therefore affect convergence—the power of the eye muscles to turn the eyes inward. Myopia may result. Adhesions of the conjunctiva of the lid to that of the eye may lead to a flattening of the cornea and hence cause hyperopia and astigmatism.

The cornea is affected by changes in curvature caused by tumors, either congenital or acquired, and also by degenerations caused by lack of specific vitamins such as vitamin A. Astigmatism is the usual result.

During its progression cataract causes changes in refraction due to the swelling of the crystalline lens. The increased curvature is evidenced by decreased hyperopia or a tendency towards myopia. Lessening power of accommodation manifests itself as premature presbyopia.

Certain congenital conditions or rare pathological involvements may cause a difference in refraction between one part of the lens and another, so that it may appear to be myopic or astigmatic in one section and hyperopic or normal in the other.

Inflammation of the bodies bordering the anterior chamber sometimes will cause an increase in the refractive index of the aqueous, because of infiltrations, and this too may manifest itself as increased myopia. Affections of the middle layer of the eye— the choroid, have been known to lead to hyperopia—particularly if there is detachment caused by injury or operation.

Forward swelling of the retina would apparently lead to hyperopia, but anterior chamber infiltrations usually supersede and indicate myopia. For that matter, any tumor or swelling that causes forward protrusion of the back of the eye globe would of necessity produce hyperopia.

The effect of glaucoma on refraction is generally considered to be an increase in hyperopia, due to poor functioning of the accommodative apparatus. But sometimes cataractous changes result which are manifested as myopia.

Any injuries—mechanical, chemical or otherwise, which alter the shape of the globe and the tissue structure of the cornea, will have an effect on refraction. The eyeball will be distorted, symptoms of astigmatism, myopia, and hyperopia will appear.

Any disturbance in external muscle balance will cause pressure on the globe and possible refractive changes.

The general structure of the bones comprising the orbit surrounding the eye will sometimes influence the growth of the eye in such a way as to induce astigmatism, or myopia or hyperopia. For the most part, this cannot be changed, but surgery can occasionally be employed to correct any serious malstructure.

There are, moreover, other maladies which may come to light during the course of a routine eye refraction. The ophthalmoscope deserves the credit for this detection, since it permits a view of the blood vessels, the media and the fundus. This is perhaps the chief ocular means by which these conditions are recognized.

We see, therefore, that many metabolic disorders may first make their appearance as refractive defects or ocular symptoms.

Modern ophthalmology is keenly aware of this and consequently properly indicated therapy is the preferred treatment rather than glasses.

Of late, myopia too has on occasion responded to specific therapy. However, this refers to myopia caused by excessive refraction of the internal crystalline lens—a result of tissue or fluid changes within the structure of the lens. The use of the drugs epinephrin or adrenalin is occasionally encouraged to reinforce a deficiency of adrenal secretion, a possible factor in progressive myopia. Thyroid insufficiency as a cause also is under investigation. And the use of vitamin D (viosterol) has been advocated to combat this form of nearsightedness as well as, in some guarded opinions, to counteract keratoconus.

Generally, the use of specific drugs, hormones or vitamins to correct refractive conditions of and by themselves has been very restricted. The chief gains of modern ophthalmology in this direction point to the inclusion in the normal diet of all known vitamins. The research which has led to these conclusions has eliminated, certainly in modern times, many borderline asthenopic (ocular discomfort) cases—where glasses were formerly accepted as the only remedy.

Exhaustive experiments have been conducted indicating a strong and elaborate correlation between proper nutrition and healthy eyesight.

Vitamin A appears to be a necessary component of the visual purple pigment layer in the back of the eye (rhodopsin) and hence its shortage slows down the formation of this essential element. Dark adaptation is impaired by a lack of vitamin A and what we know as night-blindness results.

Likewise, degenerative changes in the cornea—softening, drying and ulceration, may occur with vitamin A deprivation. Defective adaptation to dim light is frequently used as a signpost of small degrees of a lack of vitamin A, for this slight delay in dark adaptation may appear before any other symptom of vitamin A deficiency.

Since vitamin A is present in many common foods, its absence is most unusual. Carotene, the natural yellow coloring matter of many plants, including carrots and apricots, is a prime source of vitamin A, and it also is present in most green vegetables (where its color is masked by the green chlorophyll), especially in cabbage and spinach. Milk, butter, and in small amounts, eggyolk contain Carotene. Vitamin A-containing cod-liver oil, halibut-liver oil, and many liver foods are most effective in the treatment of impaired night vision.

Even the early Egyptians and Greeks were aware of this, for an Egyptian papyrus of about 1500 B.C. records it; and Hippocrates, "the Father of Medicine" (about 400 B.C.) recognized night-blindness and its cure by the administration of ox-liver.

The vitamin B series also have their place in ocular nutrition. The lack of vitamin B_1 (thiamin), in addition to leading to beri-beri, is probably the main cause of malnutritional amblyopia —a loss of vision resulting from poor nutrition. B_2 complex deficiency (riboflavin) leads to photophobia or aversion to light; B_7 (niacin) deficiency (the cause of pellagra) results in diplopia (double vision), eyelid inflammation, erosion of the eye surface tissues and clouding of the cornea . . . even paralysis of the eye muscles. Insufficient vitamin B_{12} frequently accompanies "tobacco amblyopia"—loss of vision resulting from excessive use of tobacco.

Many foods contain the B vitamins—eggs, fresh fruit, vegetables, bread, cereals, brewers' yeast, desiccated liver, wheat germ, squash seeds, sunflower seeds, nuts, pork and kidney. Like vitamin A, it too is plentiful.

Vitamin C, usually called the anti-scurvy vitamin, is equally essential for proper eye nutrition. It acts as an anti-hemorrhagic agent, by producing and maturing the substance collagen in the body. This is the cementing substance necessary for the repair of wounds and injured tissue; it makes the eye more resistant to injury.

It is possible also that vitamin C is vital to the metabolism of the crystalline lens—since it is present in an appreciable amount in the aqueous humor, the cornea and particularly in the lens cortex. From this, one might surmise that it possesses an "anti-cataract" property since its concentration here in the lens nucleus diminishes with age and with cataract formation. It is theorized that vitamin C increases the rate of oxygen absorption of the lens and thus staves off hardening of the tissue.

Vitamin C is contained in green peppers, cauliflower, broccoli, raw cabbage, strawberries, peas, tomatoes, and of course orange juice and citrus fruits.

The sunlight vitamin, D, is actually two in number, D_2 and D_3. D_2 is produced artificially by irradiating a constituent of yeast or ergot of rye with sunlight or ultraviolet light. D_3 is present in cod-liver oil and halibut-liver oil, as well as in milk, egg-yolk, butter, and other dairy products. Ordinarily it is produced directly in the skin by the action of sunlight on the fatty material secreted by the sweat glands—so its lack is very rare.

The effect on the eye is important, for its deficiency may lead to cataract, and, as previously mentioned, it is believed that because of its calcifying properties, vitamin D increases the resistance of the back portion of the sclera of the eye, reducing the tendency of the sclera to stretch. This is a cause of progressive myopia.

Vitamin E is an oxygen carrier. It facilitates the absorption and utilization of oxygen in all parts of the eye, thus easing ocular disturbances and stimulating sharpness of vision. Wheat-germ (oatmeal), rice-germ oils, green leafy vegetables such as lettuce, and in small amounts, the fat of milk—these are vitamin E's primary sources. In the drug or health-food stores it is known as the mixed tocopherols.

Vitamin K, the anti-hemorrhagic vitamin, affects the eye in much the same manner as vitamin C. It promotes blood coagulation and repair of injuries and, as far as we know, this is the only way it affects the eye's health. It is present in spinach, cabbage, cauliflower, carrot-tops, tomatoes and orange peel.

In addition to vitamins, food contains valuable eye-nutritive elements. Milk contains calcium, for instance, to clear up excessive winking or watering of the eyes, inflammation of the pigmented eye layer, conjunctivitis and photophobia. Rutin—a yellow extract of buckwheat leaves, is recommended by a famous English oculist, Dr. L. B. Somerville Large, to strengthen the eye's blood vessel walls. Proteins have been found generally beneficial in arresting eye deterioration, a cause of progressive myopia.

A theory of one American eye specialist, Dr. H. H. Turner, deplores the current popularity of carbonated beverages. He claims waterlogging of the white tissues of the eye results from excessive use and causes constriction and congestion of the blood vessels. The effect is impaired circulation, oxygen deprivation, consequent loss of visual acuity, and ocular malfunction.

The use of drugs in muscular insufficiency cases formerly correctable only by lenses or prisms, has also been advanced by research. The drug Floropryl is indicated to be of greater advantage than convex lenses. It will elicit greater accommodation. Floropryl appears to be a useful adjunct in its effect on accommodation even in cases of "amblyopia," where there is no vision at all. Atropine, used over a period of months or years, brings a degree of success in relaxing accommodation in defects such as myopia.

Also in the research stages are the uses of endocrine therapy. Pituitary tumors produce defects in the field of vision and persistent headaches. This is influenced by improper endocrine functioning prompted by liver abnormalities. Nystagmus (the involuntary oscillation of the eyes from side to side), lens opacities, and swollen eyelids may be traced to insufficiency of thyroid secretion; defective convergence is sometimes due to over-activity of the thyroid, which may also lead to thyrotoxicosis —a poisoning of the system caused by excess flow from the thyroid.

From a remedial point of view, endocrine therapy is designed to counteract these deficiencies, as well as those causing interference with the calcium fixation of the tissues enclosing the eye. This is thought to cause a constriction of the external eye muscles in near fixation and lead to a lengthening of the eyeball. This is another theory as to the causative factors of myopia.

Modern ophthalmology has further uncovered the extreme importance psychosomatic effects occupy in both refractive error and the apparent resultant eyestrain.

Hyperopia, astigmatism and muscular anomalies most frequently give rise to eyestrain. Yet when the degree of defect is small it is difficult to ascertain how much of the eyestrain or ocular discomfort is due to the defect and how much to the emotional and psychological state of the sufferer. Studies of this problem point preponderantly to the greater role played by the latter condition.

Hypochondriasis—the preoccupation of the individual with his bodily functions and dysfunctions, leads to inordinate symptoms of eyestrain.

Frustration at near work . . . reading page upon page of dull material . . . boredom when the eyes are employed at monotonous tasks . . . are readily understood to provoke a complaint of eyestrain. The strain is promptly relieved if the particular chore is made more interesting.

The emotional state of the individual and, of course, his general physical state can lead to reduced energy and lessened well-being, inevitably giving rise to eye symptoms ordinarily too minor to be troublesome.

Even cases of myopia of accepted structural origin, and certainly myopia of muscular or tonic origin (called pseudomyopia), can be attributed to inhibition and repression of normal visual curiosity stemming, in some cases, from profound psychological withdrawal and introversion. Whether the withdrawal from the environment results from the myopia or vice versa, there no doubt is a decided link between the two.

In properly diagnosing these and other effects, the role of psychotherapy has assumed increasing importance in the modern refractionist's regimen. Referring these individuals for medical or psychiatric care rather than refractive correction has in many cases eliminated the need for sight correction.

In the heightened understanding of the part proper light and color plays in visual (and even systemic) disturbances lies the improvements in modern conditions which similarly lessen the need for refractive correction.

Studies have shown that red colors, for instance, are stimulating and warm, green shades relaxing and cool. Some hospitals have found that a blue room acts as a sedative for some patients:

psychiatric hospitals have used this knowledge for violent inmates. Yellow, on the other hand, may be quite disturbing, even nausea-producing—one reason airlines shun its use in the interior decor of aircraft. Yellow foods, people discover, should be avoided during sea or air travel.

Similarly, color apparently will change the temperature. A blue room appears cool and may even cause occupants to feel chilly; an orange room gives the sensation of sunlight and warmth, although the actual temperature may be identical in both cases.

The effect of color on weight is interesting. Dark objects will appear heavier, light ones lighter. Moreover, our judgment of time may be influenced by color. Most people overestimate the passage of time when surrounded by red, and underestimate it when surrounded by green or blue. Hence one hour may seem like two under red surroundings, and two like one under green.

So far as the eyes are concerned, red colors definitely stimulate their reflexes, green relaxes them. For this reason, and because blue colors reduce blood pressure and induce relaxation, green or blue are desirable bedroom colors.

Light and color engineering has made definite contributions to more efficient use of the eyes, and to lessened dependency on border-line refractive conditions.

Improved hygiene, both personal and public, are obvious advancements in the same direction.

The role of surgery, too, must not be overlooked in relation to the eye's refraction. Probably the major forms of eye surgery deal with the refractive media of the eye—the crystalline lens and the cornea, as well as the muscular defects affecting the refractive error. And the advances in eye surgery, including these forms, have been great within recent times.

Without doubt the most classic condition requiring eye surgery for a media obstruction is a cataract, where vision is obscured by a milky-white film within the pupil.

The name is derived from medieval Latin translations of Arabic writings, which describe it as "humor flowing down into the eye." It refers to what was understood to be a collection of opaque matter formed between the pupil and the lens.

The writings of an ancient Greek physician, Celsus, give a detailed account of both the medical and the pre- and post-operative treatment. A later Roman writer attributed the operative procedure to the casual observation that vision was restored to a goat, blind from cataract, when it ran its eye onto a thorn.

Not until the 18th century was this concept—opaque matter deposited between the lens and pupil—disproven as the cause of cataract, and the true source of cataract—opacification of the lens itself—established.

About 1,000 years ago an Arab surgeon devised the procedure of piercing a soft lens with a hollow needle and sucking out enough material to remove the impediment to sight.

In 1748 the French physician Daviel published his account of the extraction of the cataractous lens. Formerly, "couching" the lens was practiced. This constituted breaking the opaque material into smaller pieces with a needle and causing it to crumble and be displaced into another part of the eye, usually the vitreous chamber.

It was the unplanned displacement of the lens into the aqueous chamber that started Daviel on his planned extraction of the entire lens. Present-day intracapsular extractions (from within the capsule enveloping the lens) were made possible by the developments in local anaesthesia—but not until the late 19th century, when the work of eye surgeons von Graefe and Mooren contributed heavily.

Modern-day cataract surgery is responsible for the restoration of useful sight to many eyes, and has become an operative procedure almost as routine as tonsillectomy and appendectomy. Lens extraction causes the eye to become very far-sighted, because approximately 13 diopters of power are eliminated. A strong convex lens must then be applied in order to bring images into proper focus.

During recent years an important adjunct of the cataract

extraction operation has been the utilization of the so-called anterior chamber lenses to replace the extracted lens. This is a tiny, bean-shaped, all-plastic acrylic lens, fabricated in powers ranging from nine to fourteen diopters and in diameters from ten to fourteen millimeters.

Prof. Harold Ridley of London, in 1952, introduced this ingenious method of circumventing the necessity for wearing a thick cataract spectacle lens. Immediately after removing the opaque lens from its capsule, he inserted into the capsule a tiny, plastic lens conforming in size and shape to the average, human adult lens. The patient may have to wear ordinary low power lenses over them to get best acuity and to correct the astigmatism created by cutting through the cornea.

When this unorthodox operation was described, a new field in operative research of the eyes was opened. Later, in 1954, an Italian ophthalmologist, Dr. B. Strampelli, modified Ridley's technique by placing the acrylic lens into the anterior chamber.

One form of this lens, Fig. 38, has what is called peripheral loop mounts—flexible resilient plastic mounts which collapse when the lens is implanted and then spring open to serve as anchorage when it is in place.

Two to three months after a cataract operation this implantation is performed. Experimental results have been guardedly successful. It is reported that implantation can be used in all

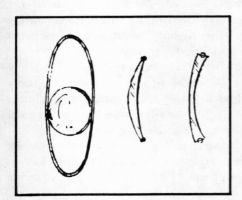

Fig. 38: The anterior chamber lens with collapsible mounts. (Titmus Optical)

types of cataract surgery, as long as no complications are involved. There are, however, certain contraindications present in a minority of cases.

Visual results, in the limited number of cases reported, are encouraging: 18 of 29 show acuity of 20/25 or better with an additional spectacle correction of only plus or minus 2 diopters. In the remaining 11, visual acuity was comparable to or slightly better than the corrected vision of the eye before implantation. In no case was vision poorer than that with conventional lenses.

Experimental studies in cases of high myopia and hyperopia have been carried out in the use of the anterior chamber lens. Sometimes performed monocularly—to correct a great degree of difference between the two eyes, and sometimes binocularly—to improve vision jointly, results in 28 such cases have produced vision the same or better than by other means.

During the eighteenth and nineteenth centuries, too, tentative attempts were made to relieve loss of vision resulting from opacities of the cornea. As early as 1795 an English physician, Erasmus Darwin, trephined (sectioned) out opaque areas of the cornea, hoping to obtain clear areas on healing. And the problem of complete transplantation of the cornea attracted much attention during the first third of the next century.

Though successful experimentally in rabbits, corneal transplantation at this time failed in man. Even the idea of implanting a small glass lens in the cornea, offered in 1856, was not successful. Only recently has it been recognized that corneal transplanting (called keratoplasty) can succeed only when it is partial—not total, and when the grafted material is of human origin.

Modern eye banks, which preserve healthy corneas for transplanting, exist throughout the world. In many cases such a transplant will restore visual acuity close to normal, replacing a scarred or nebulous cornea with one perfectly clear and regular in curvature. In others refractive assistance is necessary.

In this connection, it is interesting to note that intracapsular tests have shown that the opaque cornea does not truly lose its light-transmitting powers but simply becomes translucent rather than transparent. An image is therefore formed on the cornea similar to the ground glass of a camera.

The possibility of using this ground glass effect is suggested by replacing both the crystalline lens with an acrylic lens within the lens capsule and also inserting a second acrylic lens in the anterior chamber. Together they may serve to project the corneal picture on the retina—provided the refractive power is adequate. And although it is hardly likely the limited refracting power of present-day acrylic lenses (1.5) is adequate even in combination, other materials with higher indexes—crystalline materials such as strontium titanate (2.409), rutile titanium dioxide (2.613), antimony sulfate (3), or higher index—may very well be produced.

Unquestionably such methods, with artificial intraocular lenses of high refractive index may bring light and sight to many otherwise incurably blind persons, no matter how clumsy or primitive the sight may be.

Even iridectomies (incisions in the iris) were tried in order to bring a clear part of the scarred or nebulous cornea into the line of vision, but for the most part these are now limited to certain pathological conditions.

Another form of surgery sometimes utilized in cases of ocular difficulty is that involving severance of certain sensory eye nerves —chiefly to relieve intractable pain. This has limited application, and its use, moreover, in migraine pain—that inexplicable and chronic pain which has eluded cure for centuries, has not proven satisfactory.

During the course of surgery for retinal detachment (a condition occurring in some cases of high myopia where there is extreme elongation and stretching of the eyeball) shortening of the eyeball has been accomplished by excision of parts of the sclera at the point of retinal detachment.

In 10 of 21 patients with whom this was employed, satisfactory results were produced—namely retinal reattachment, and, from the point of view of refraction, reduction of the myopia. At present the use of this radical surgery for reduction of myopia alone is contra-indicated. In a few desperate cases of extreme myopia a thin strip of sclera has been cut away—decreasing the size of the globe and allowing the retina to fit better into the smaller space.

Insofar as the muscular defects are concerned, the field of surgery has made enormous strides.

The nineteenth century immeasurably advanced the treatment of squint, or crossed-eyes—the result of muscular defects.

Known but vaguely understood in antiquity, squint was always the "evil eye" of mythology and primitive folklore. In the writings of Hippocrates, the father of medicine, it is clearly recognized that squint frequently affects both parents and children.

An early attempt at treatment was made in the seventh century by a Byzantine physician, Paulus Aegineta, and is the first recorded effort. He had a patient wear a mask with two perforations placed centrally before the eyes. Only by looking directly ahead, it was argued, could the squinting eye see through the opening. Fixing bright objects to the outer side of an inturning eye was likewise attempted; this, it was held, would excite attention and make the turning eye assume a normal position.

During the eighteenth century, squint was still regarded as the result of malposition of the cornea or a tilting of the eye's crystalline lens. Not until an itinerant French practitioner, Chevalier Taylor, discovered its correlation with the external muscles of the eye and performed division of the affected muscle (tenotomy) which produced straightening, were these beliefs revised.

One hundred years later, in 1827, orthodox practitioners were suggesting this type of operation for squint, and in 1839 the first successful such operation was performed by the German physician Dieffenbach.

Numerous modifications have followed to this day, but essentially the operation remains the same. It is a relatively harmless one, since it does not involve the interior of the eye at all. In most cases the squint is due to a shortened muscle which has drawn the eyeball in its direction. The surgeon simply separates the muscle from its attachment to the eyeball and resutures it to another part farther back. This permits the eye to straighten. In some cases the muscle may be too long, therefore allowing the eye to turn away from it. Here the surgeon shortens the muscle in order to tighten its control of the eyeball. (Likening these muscles to the reins used to direct the turning of a horse's head, is a very apt comparison. A shorter rein must be loosened or let slack, a longer rein tightened, in order for the horse's head to be directed forward.)

Moreover, modern research has shown that certain squint cases can be corrected without surgery or only partially with surgery. Dating from the mid-19th century, theories of fusion—the innate desire of the eyes to work together—and of correlation between the muscles controlling accommodation (focusing for near vision) and convergence (turning of the eyes together for near vision) have led to other measures for the treatment and control of squint. Simultaneously they have led to other explorations which touch on the neuro-muscular and psychological attributes of vision.

Eye exercises is the catch-all phrase used to label these explorations.

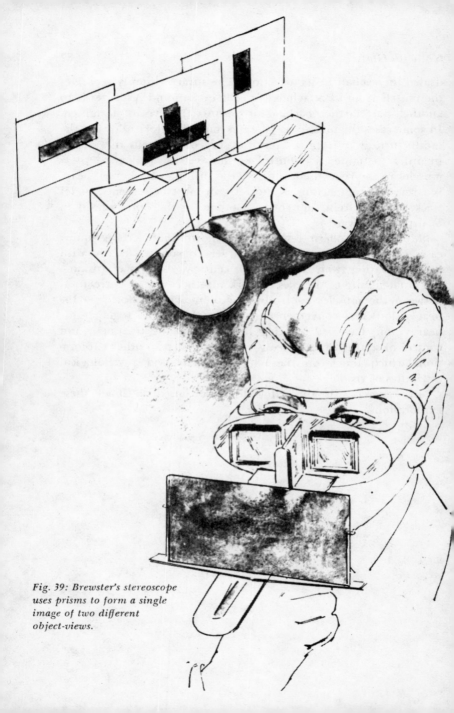

Fig. 39: Brewster's stereoscope uses prisms to form a single image of two different object-views.

VII

The Value of Eye Exercises

With the principles of Paulus Aegineta pointing the way, it became common practice in later years to cover or occlude the normal eye in cases of squint. This compelled the defective, turned eye to work and develop normal vision—absent in a turned eye. It was believed that the eye turned because of this vision lack, and this was confirmed in many cases since the eye straightened when vision was improved.

A French oculist, duBois-Raymond, expressed the basic theories of this form of eye exercise. His beliefs were initially propounded around 1850; they were further elaborated upon by Javal before the end of the century. Javal's research on the nature of fusion—the inherent urge for the two eyes to fuse into one the image seen by each—provided the foundation for modern-day orthoptic training, the accepted name by which orthodox eye training is called today.

Javal proved, and was later supported by the English physician Claud Worth, that fusion—the single binocular viewing of an object—was the natural state of the eyes, and that only when they are prevented from assuming this state—by pathological causes (muscle paralysis), nerve involvements, or refractive defects—is fusion lost and a squint developed.

The invention of the streoscope by Wheatstone in 1838 provided the impetus for the detailed research in ensuing years which led to and confirmed Javal's and Worth's theories. Further it led to methods for correcting defects of fusion.

The great advantage of fusion—and apparently nature's purpose for developing it in higher forms of life, is that it permits depth perception—tri-dimensional or "stereoscopic" vision. Both eyes, because of the slightly different angle of viewing, do not see an object in exactly the same way.

Figure 40 shows that if a three-dimensional object, such as a pencil, is held directly facing the bridge of the nose, the right eye will see it from one aspect, the left eye from another.

These so-called disparate images are unified by the mind into one perceptual image. Thus, the pencil is seen as a solid body. If there were no retinal disparity a three-dimensional object would appear flat—having no depth or solidity.

Wheatstone employed this principle in creating an instrument, shown in Fig. 41, which allowed each eye to see pictures of an object taken from the angle the eye would have made with the object. In other words, two photographs were taken—one as the right eye would see an object—the other as seen by the left eye. These two photographs were then mounted in the so-called stereoscope; with the use of mirrors, as illustrated, the proper image pertaining to each eye was viewed by that eye.

Shortly thereafter, Brewster, another English scientist, improved the Wheatstone idea by substituting prisms for the mirrors (Fig. 39). This achieved the same effect and was a great deal easier on the viewer since the eyes converge naturally, instead of looking straight ahead.

In recent years other variations of instruments designed to produce stereoscopic effects have appeared. Since their chief purpose is to permit two slightly differing images to be viewed by the two eyes, other means of accomplishing this have been devised. If one picture is printed in red, for instance, and the other picture in green, a red glass in front of one eye will permit only the red picture to be seen, and a green glass in front of the other will permit only the green light to pass. Not long ago the rage of 3-D motion pictures was based purely on this effect, and, if the reader recalls, red-green filters were utilized by the viewer.

The same effect is achieved by polaroid filters—used exten-

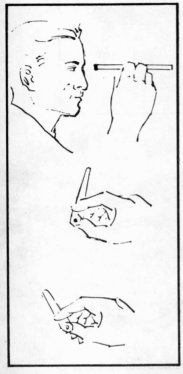

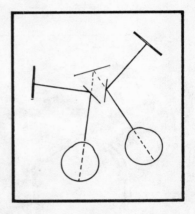

Fig. 40: The right eye sees one view, the left another. Both are fused to give the perception of depth.

Fig. 41: Wheatstone's stereoscope used mirrors to view different photographs of the same object.

sively in home stereoscopic exercises, filtering the light polarized in one plane for one eye and polarized in another plane for the other eye.

By its nature, the stereoscope made binocular vision very obvious when it was present, and it became a very important diagnostic tool in determining the prevalence of fusion. Claud Worth advanced its value in this direction by a modification of this instrument—his amblyoscope.

The amblyoscope (Fig. 42) held two entirely dissimilar objects (rather than the same one from different angles), such as a picture of a bird before one eye and the picture of a cage before the other. This immediately revealed which, if either, eye had suppressed or amblyopic vision.

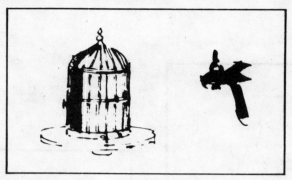

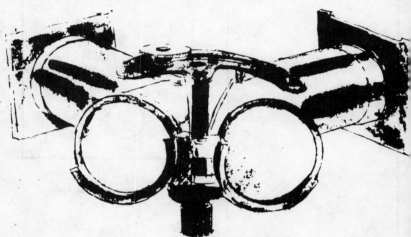

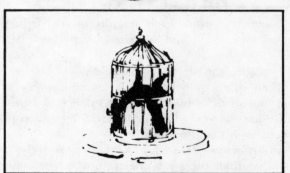

Fig. 42: A different object is viewed by each eye. Prior familiarity awakens the desire to fuse their images into one.

In the course of training, the principle of occlusion was first applied: the good eye completely blacked out and only the defective eye permitted to see. With high illumination and flashing illumination, the vision in this eye was gradually stimulated until an image was perceived, even when the other eye was uncovered. The patient would then attempt—with the help of prisms if the eye were badly turned, to bring the two images together, so that the bird would be inside the cage.

Practically all orthoptic instruments in use today are modelled after the Worth amblyoscope. All are based on the premise 1) of awakening or stimulating vision in the deviating eye, 2) rendering assistance to it in the form of prisms to encourage fusion with its mate, and 3) gradually reducing the strength of these prisms as the muscle tone of the eye improves and the stimulus to fusion suffices to maintain single vision.

In addition, modern research has raised other interesting points: in some cases, squint is tied to a refractive error.

Donders, in 1864, showed the presence of high hyperopia in certain cases of convergent squint. He pointed out that there appeared to be a link between the excess accommodative effort needed to overcome the hyperopia and the excess convergence effort evident in the squint. Moreover, he applied convex lenses to correct the hyperopia and immediately found that the squint disappeared.

Today, this type of squint—called accommodative squint—has become the easiest to correct. All that is needed is the proper refractive correction, and this a farsighted one.

In a divergent squint (wall-eye), it might appear logical to tie this to lessened accommodative effort (allied to nearsightedness) and to attempt to correct this by stimulating accommodation by concave lenses—thus increasing convergence. Generally, however, this is not successful, and only surgery is of value.

Another fact modern research has brought to light is that squint, in truth, is a two-faced problem: one manifest—as in the cases of eyes that turn, and the other latent—in cases where the tendency for the eyes to turn is overcome by excessive neuro-muscular effort. This effort leads to many of the newly-recognized symptoms of eyestrain, and, in this connection, properly applied training serves to correct the improper tendency.

Perhaps the chief offender in this category is what is called convergence insufficiency—where the muscles converging the eyes are inadequate to their task. Symptoms of eyestrain result which, in previous years, led to wearing eyeglasses frequently quite ineffectual.

To correct this insufficiency by strengthening the muscles, a simple exercise can be employed with a pencil—a good illustration of what more intricate exercises seek to improve. If a pencil is held approximately 25 inches from the face and then brought closer to the nose, the eye will exert effort to focus and to maintain a single image by turning inward. With exercising, moving the pencil back and forth repeatedly, it will be found possible to approach the nose closer and closer before a doubling—signifying a loss of binocular vision—occurs.

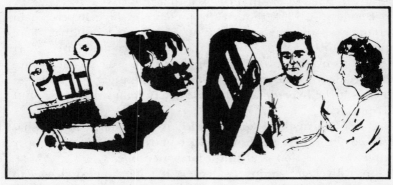

Fig. 43A and 43B: Two instruments commonly used to exercise the eye muscles.

There is, of course, a normal "near point" of convergence where normal eyes cannot maintain single binocular vision—a point approximately six inches away depending upon age and other factors. Any inability to reach this is considered a convergence insufficiency. Rarely is there a hyperactivity of convergence, and this generally points to a source of infection somewhere.

When instruments are used—usually the "telebinocular" or

"stereo-orthopter," they employ prisms in graduated steps which force the convergent muscles to become more and more active in order to maintain single binocular vision. Later on, home exercises in addition to the pencil exercise are employed. Special training cards—polaroid and red-green as well as the stereoscope, are utilized, first to create a stereoscopic effect fostering fusion, and second to make fusion more difficult calling for increased convergent effort to maintain it.

"Bar reading"—holding a pencil or other object in front of the face and approximately in the line of sight while reading— is encouraged since part of the reading matter will be obscured from either eye. This reveals if and when one eye suppresses vision, i.e., gives up in its attempt to participate in binocular vision.

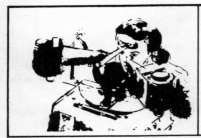 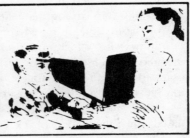

Fig. 43C: The "troposcope" is another instrument utilizing prism variations.

Fig. 43D: The bar separator which prevents an overlapping of images.

Aside from the application of orthoptics to straightening the eyes—both pre-operatively and post-operatively to promote more satisfactory fusion, and its use in strengthening unused or inadequate muscles, there remains the question of whether "exercises" eliminate or reduce the need for refractive correction.

The close relationship Donders cited between the accommodation and the convergence has been elaborated and expanded to the point where, some modern practitioners feel, anything affecting the accommodation will affect convergence and vice versa.

The logical conclusion of this—not wholly borne out by clinical fact, would be that any excess accommodative effort—such as that producing functional myopia, could be relieved, not by supplying concave lenses (which is standard procedure in myopia) but by advising prism exercises (base in) to relax the convergence and thus relax the accommodation.

By the same token, certain modern theories hold that myopia is the result of an inherent weakness of the convergent muscles, calling for extra nervous effort in order to turn the eyes inward for near vision. This extra effort will have its effect on the accommodative muscles, causing them too to become over-stimulated. Because of this the focusing of the eye's lens is increased and the total refraction of the eye becomes greater. In some cases this accounts for the total myopia of the individual; in others the inherent structural myopia increases.

Exercises to strengthen the convergent muscles (again the use of prisms in graduated steps) will lessen the need for additional nervous effort and therefore relieve the accommodative overactivity. The success or failure of this type of therapy is still open to question, but there are reported cases of virtual elimination of low grade myopia resulting from it.

Other methods used in the "cure" of myopia are similarly based on the theory of excessive accommodative effort. The sometime-recommended practice of undercorrecting nearsighted glasses is designed to allow this excess effort to subside. The use of bifocals or highly undercorrected concave lenses for reading in the case of myopic individuals carries this principle further—in the sense of actually forcing the accommodation to relax in order to preserve clarity of vision. The effect is the same as a convex lens—namely, to inhibit focusing. In fact, convex lenses will sometimes be prescribed even for nearsightedness for exactly this purpose. Results are just as questionable here as when prisms are used.

The usefulness of orthoptics in other refractive errors is primarily linked to its vision-stimulating qualities. Hyperopia and astigmatism are not even hypothesized as correctable by prism or other exercises. But more advanced stages of farsightedness or astigmatism, as well as myopia, are benefited by orthoptics. These stages are called amblyopia, or a loss of useful vision due to non-use of the eye—sometimes occasioned by a high, uncorrected refractive error.

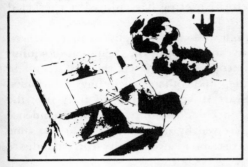

Fig. 44: The "cheiroscope" coordinates hand and eye.

Orthoptics applied to these cases seeks to stimulate vision, just as it does in squint, and then to promote fusion. Flashing lights illuminating large targets of fixation are employed. Gradually the targets are reduced in size and the speed of flashing slowed, so that the amblyopic eye is forced to retain the image longer. Form, color and movement of the target are varied to promote awakening of vision, of interest, and of intensification of perception.

In many cases the individual is encouraged to engage in physical activities to associate the act of seeing with other senses. For instance, he may be asked to hop or to step on selected squares or colored strips of cardboard; to string colored beads, or stick colored pins into selected letters of the alphabet. Occasionally an instrument such as the cheiroscope (Fig. 44) may be used. This is an ingenious device which compels the individual to trace the picture viewed by his defective eye by projecting it on a tablet. Thus his interpretative powers are improved and what was once a retinal blur gradually assumes more familiar outlines. His responsiveness to refractive correction is heightened and, in some cases, reduction of strength of glasses needed can be accomplished.

However, here is where the chief splitting-off occurs between what is considered orthodox visual training—orthoptics, and unorthodox—so-called eye exercises designed to eliminate glasses. Precisely where the psychological element comes into play is where this takes place. And the use of various types of eye exercises to eliminate refractive error has enjoyed a checkered career.

In 1896 Priestly Smith, a well-known English oculist, utilized a psychological or educative approach to the treatment of squint. Claud Worth, of amblyoscope fame, started the first clinic in London for this training, and others, including the famed ophthalmologist, Sir Stewart Duke-Elder, probed fully into the physiological theories of binocular vision, retinal correspondence (the identity of images received by the two eyes from the same object) and anomalous correspondence (faulty correspondence due to a turn in the eye).

From the work of these men—which furthered the treatment of squint and the growth of orthoptics—it was but a short step to the efforts of both medical and nonmedical practitioners at the turn of the century to use eye exercises in an attempt to avoid the need for eye-glasses.

In its most extreme form this mode of visual correction was originally propounded by Dr. William H. Bates, a New York oculist, early in this century. The school of thought he created has acquired quite a history and taken unto itself many devotees.

Dr. Bates' theory, admirably simple, was that nearsightedness, farsightedness and astigmatism were caused by abnormal actions of the six external eye muscles. Overcontraction of some muscles produced nearsightedness; of others produced farsightedness or astigmatism. And, his theory held, these conditions were forced and temporary, and could always be made to disappear by exercises directed primarily at the patient's psychological state.

In their simplicity, Dr. Bates' theories maintained that all glasses could be discarded if strain and tension were eliminated. To attain this he evolved a series of exercises pertinent to the type of strain or tension experienced. His followers and disciples have since expanded and elaborated these exercises.

He proposed that some individuals could relieve certain

tensions by staring at a blank wall, others could achieve this end by controlling thoughts or thinking pleasant thoughts.

Palming (placing the palms of both hands over the eyes to conjure up the image of black, a color purported to have corrective and healing powers) was still another technique. Once perfect black is seen, according to Dr. Bates' philosophy, perfect relaxation is attained and eyesight is restored to normal. Completely disregarded, however, is the fact that physiologically speaking, the healthy eye never sees black. Luminous sensation, caused by mechanical pressure of the blood vessels against retinal cells and other factors, is always present.

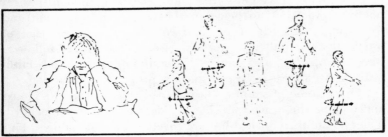

Fig. 45A: "Palming" as recommended by Bates.

Fig. 45B: The "Long Swing."

Memory and imagination—memory of a perfect black, imagination of an absolute black—these too were part of his creed.

Shifting the eyes to counteract that bane of good sight—staring—was one of the exercises. The so-called long swing—swaying the body from side to side slowly and easily to relax the eyes, the mind, the spine and the back of the neck (Fig. 45B), and the short swing—swaying only the head to relax the nerves and muscles to the back of the head and neck (Fig. 46A), were also recommended.

Both these exercises purportedly have their effect in promoting proper circulation and relaxation for the eyes. They are performed with the eyes closed, so that in essence they are concerned with mental relaxation and visualization. Suggestion is given as to the proper thoughts and imagery to accompany

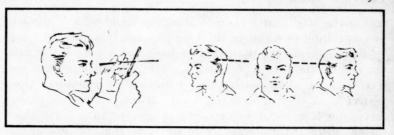

Fig. 46A: The "Short Swing."   Fig. 46B: Moving the cross-stick
                                      to and fro purportedly
                                      straightens the eyes.

these exercises—preferably the most pleasant thoughts, of a hobby or vacation, to heighten the feeling of relaxation and well-being. Evidently these represent a multiple marriage of osteopathic manipulative procedure (some of Dr. Bates' followers were osteopaths) and suggestion, auto-suggestion, and faith-healing. All appear to be essential for proper Bates training.

The exercise of sunning—facing the sun with the eyes closed and moving the head from side to side, was also recommended. The eyes are then opened but are covered with the palms. (This process theoretically possessed healing qualities!) Looking directly at the sun with the eyes opened and uncovered follows—contrary to a negative consensus of ophthalmological opinion. To support the benefits of this exercise, cases are cited of individuals suffering from photophobia who were allegedly cured by sunning!

The Bates method for correcting squint should not be overlooked. Figure 46B shows the greatly simplified training which supposedly remedies this condition. A stick is held in a position directly outward from the bridge of the nose and is used as a line upon which a pencil is drawn toward and away from the nose. The proper viewing of an X or V, after repeated attempts, will indicate that simultaneous fusion is occurring in both eyes.

Of course, these exercises are frowned upon and disavowed by practically all trained eye practitioners, because of Bates' complete disregard of sound physiological principles—the confirmed theories of accommodation, refraction and muscular activity.

Perhaps the only instance in which the Bates method approaches accepted therapy is in its stress of general bodily health, particularly good posture. In all other respects it is completely at odds with orthodox ocular therapy and orthoptics.

Without question, the strongest reason why Bates' system apparently produces some success lies in the encouragement and confidence the exercises can give a psychoneurotic individual. The person emotionally insecure in his ability to see, tensed by fear of the danger of using his eyes, gains relaxation, confidence, reassurance and a feeling of empathy with his teacher.

Basically, one can not deny that the effect of relaxation on tensed muscles, however taught, is a beneficial one, and here too is the principal value of this type of eye exercise.

Though there are many failures among would-be Bates method students (attributed by advocates to the lack of perseverance), there are, to be sure, a fair number of gratified graduates who apparently have discarded their glasses. A simple psychological explanation in addition to the emotional climate described, is probably the best answer.

The Bates method subscribes to the theory that sight is nine-tenths mental and only one-tenth physical. Simple exercises to think about what you see, to visualize only small areas at a time, to avoid concentrated fixation or staring, to keep shifting the eyes frequently, and to blink often—these are the prime requisites of not only comfortable eyesight but normal eyesight as well.

And these methods are not far removed from the psychological approach to vision we mentioned earlier as marking the separation between orthoptics and other eye exercises.

It has been demonstrated that many people can be taught to interpret blurred images more efficiently so that they learn to read more letters on the Snellen chart. Thus, a learning process—rather than a corrective process—is employed. It is quite possible to take any cooperative individual, and, with suitable instruments or even suggestion, increase his ability to interpret imperfect or too-small retinal images. Practice of and by itself in interpreting images leads to improvement. For example, a seaman will recognize an image in the distance as a vessel, while a landlubber may only see a blur. The sailor has trained himself to see beyond the blur—and this actually enables him to perceive more fully the outlines of an approaching ship.

That this improvement does not persist beyond a recognition of more or less familiar objects, is well proven by a case reported by publisher Bennett Cerf in the *Saturday Review,* April 12, 1952.

The famed British author, Aldous Huxley, had for a long time boasted that eye exercises had restored his sight to normal. He had written extensively on the subject; his was a prime example of what eye exercises could do *(The Art of Seeing).*

At 16 he had had a violent inflammation of the cornea which, after 18 months of near blindness, left one eye just capable of light perception and the other eye with a vision of 20/200. Correcting lenses brought vision up to about 20/100 and with the aid of a hand magnifier he took up again his interrupted college course and graduated from Oxford University.

His near vision became increasingly worse and more fatiguing, and he was afraid he would soon not be able to read at all. At this point, instead of seeking medical advice and application of the visual aids available at that time (1939) Mr. Huxley threw all recognized professional and scientific ophthalmic work overboard and embarked on an adventure of visual exercises.

In his book, Mr. Huxley purports to show how he has improved his vision without recourse to glasses, but purely by a series of eye- and mind-exercises. He makes the claim that all visual defects can be greatly alleviated without the use of glasses but merely by the application of the exercises he describes.

On one particular occasion, Mr. Cerf was listening to Huxley give a prepared address, impressed by the fact that this man, once on the threshold of blindness, could now read without glasses. Suddenly Huxley faltered. Cerf realized that the novelist was not really reading his manuscript. Rather, he had attempted to memorize it. Huxley brought his eyes closer and closer to the printed page.

Finally, in despair, he took a magnifying glass from his pocket to make the words readable. Cerf describes the episode as one of agony. . . .

Evidently Huxley used to the utmost the very limited vision he possessed . . . this shows to what an extent will and motivation can overcome the handicap of a poorly and partly functioning eye.

Still another glaring proof of the limited value of the psychological approach is the fact that so many Bates practitioners themselves wear glasses!

~~⊙⊙~~

Educative processes have also been used to improve color recognition. Color-blind or near-color-blind servicemen have been helped by study via the "Ishihara Color Tests." Though still technically color-blind, they were able after repeated sessions of studying and identifying the charts, to recognize certain visual stimuli in terms of color—purely a learning process.

The application of eye exercises to reading disabilities is a frank acknowledgement of the educative and psychological approach, rather than a refractive or therapeutic one.

Here the types of exercises used—while engaging the eyes in activity, are primarily concerned with teaching the proper perception and interpretation of visual impressions. Properly speaking they are not really eye exercises, since it is not the eyes at all which are exercised, but rather the ability to grasp and retain images which is fostered. As a matter of fact, it is frequently found that poor reading ability is present with extremely good and comfortable visual acuity, and that better than average reading ability and comprehension is not unusual in cases of below-normal vision.

The fact that educational surveys indicate that 15 to 25% of the school-age population has some degree of reading difficulty shows the increasing importance of this facet of visual utilization. Generally, these surveys will disclose that reading skill lags behind other scholastic achievements, that numbers and musical notes are read more easily than words, that letters of certain words may be reversed (felt read as left), that writing words from dictation is laborious and, in general, there is a lack of word comprehension.

Only a small proportion of these difficulties is due to visual problems. Most are due to poor educational training, hearing or emotional problems, reversed left- or right-handedness, glandular deficiencies, congenital or inherited defects and other conditions beyond the scope of eye therapy.

The institution of remedial reading classes in many clinics and schools—alongside classes in visual rehabilitation and sight conservation—is meeting the problem as it should be met, on an educational rather than therapeutic level. And although eye instruments are used in some cases (such as the tachistoscope, Fig. 47)—to increase the span of reading and word recognition by timed illumination of cards, it must be repeated that remedial reading is not eye exercises.

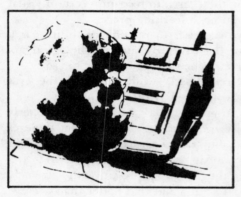

Fig. 47: The "tachistoscope" regulates reading speed by timed exposure of words.

Apart from the application of psychological eye exercises, there is no doubt that accredited, fully-substantiated orthoptic exercises have their great value in ameliorating or eliminating ocular difficulties. In some cases they will lead to the discarding of eye-glasses. Certainly this can be expected to increase, as what are labelled refractive difficulties are more properly identified as neuro-muscular difficulties amenable to correction by properly applied exercises.

Unfortunately, however, most refractive difficulties rest on a firm basis of structural defect and so we must look to other means of correction.

VIII

The Neglected Blind

Do errors of refraction ever lead to blindness?

This provocative question, though usually unspoken, is frequently present in the mind of the individual who suffers from a high visual defect.

It is a question which has two answers, and it depends on what we consider blindness.

If, on the one hand, we think of blindness in the traditional sense—the total and complete inability to distinguish light from dark, the answer is an unqualified "no."

There has never been a recorded case of refractive error, regardless of degree, corrected or uncorrected, known to cause blindness. No loss of visual acuity due to lack of proper refraction has ever led to blindness; and, conversely, proper refraction which might restore normal visual acuity has not of itself prevented ultimate blindness originating from other causes.

The absolute blindness we speak of has, from ancient times, been known to result from many causes—none of them refractive in nature. Blindness has been caused by injuries, accidental or otherwise.

Galen's theory of corrupt humors explains loss of vision as the result of a flow of secretions, or injurious spirits, from the brain to various parts of the eye. When this secretion flowed to the crystalline lens, it caused the lens to lose moisture. This gave the eye a greenish discoloration, to which the name glaucoma was given. To this day, glaucoma remains a principal cause of blindness.

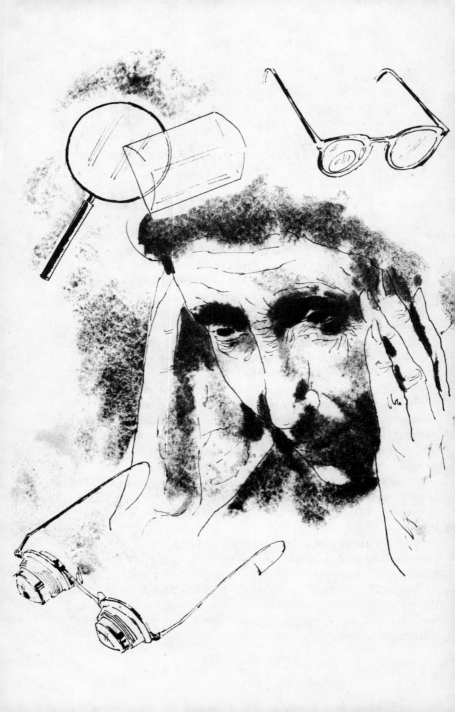

When the spirits settled in front of the crystalline lens, it collected between the pupil and the lens and obstructed vision. The condition was called a cataract.

Of the two, glaucoma invariably resulted in blindness—no cure or remedy was known until much later. Cataract responded in limited fashion to medication and couching, but remains to this day a very significant cause of blindness.

Ocular hemorrhages, external diseases such as trachoma (the highly-contagious and dangerous lid infection which is the scourge of Egypt, India and China), and inflammations of the eye surfaces, were observed and understood, even in ancient times, to lead to blindness. Unfortunately, awareness did not produce remedies.

Diseases affecting the interior of the eye were not recognized. These included the iris, the ciliary body (structures surrounding the iris and crystalline lens), the innermost layers of the eye, the retina and the choroid (the middle layer between the retina and the outside sclera).

Involvements of the optic nerve and its extensions—or of the brain itself—as causes for blindness, these were not even dreamed about.

Not until 1818 when the English physician, Wardrop, published his "Essays on the Morbid Anatomy of the Human Eye," did the modern trend of thinking develop on the origin and causes of blindness as we have defined it.

By this time cataract had already been properly identified and treatment achieved some degree of success. Glaucoma, however, remained incurable until late in the nineteenth century, when its cause was accurately ascribed to an "increase in fluid tension inside the eye." Excess intraocular fluid and improper drainage, it was discovered, led to increased pressure on the inside walls of the eye, impairment of circulation and ultimate deterioration of vision. Absolute blindness was invariably the result.

With the increase in anti-infective measures during the early twentieth century, many of the external ocular diseases were brought under control. Their effect diminished as causes of blindness. Intra-ocular affections: iritis, iridocyclitis, choroiditis and retinitis were recognized and treatment devised. Corneal inflammations such as keratitis, and their aftereffects, became amenable to cure. Nerve involvements, brain lesions and tumors, were diagnosed.

The gradual impairment of vision resulting from organic malfunction in some cases led to blindness. In other instances the impairment was arrested by proper therapy. Cataract surgery and treatment made remarkable advances. Even glaucoma, the dread disease of centuries, responded to therapy and surgery.

Gradually the incidence of absolute blindness diminished. True, each affection left its mark. Lid diseases left their mark in scars and distortions. Corneal inflammations would scar, roughen and opacify certain corneal areas. But iris operations would reduce the effect of iritis, cataract surgery would minimize lens opacities. Retinal reattachment and therapy would modify the previously calamitous effect of detachment or retinitis, leaving only isolated areas of damaged or atrophied nerve cells.

And it was found that light sensation was still present and fleeting images could still be seen.

Blindness had taken on a new dimension.

It was no longer the complete and total absence of light sensation—such as severing the optic nerve might produce, but a variable degree of sensitivity due at times only to localized damage to nerve cells of the retina or to localized obstructions in the various eye media.

Even the definition of blindness changed. According to the U.S. Department of Health, Education and Welfare, blindness today is defined as "vision insufficient for the ordinary activities of life for which sight is required." Ophthalmologically speaking, this means "central visual acuity not exceeding 20/200 (Snellen) in the better eye with correction; or central visual acuity greater than 20/200 but accompanied by a limitation of the fields of vision by 20 degrees."

In these cases blindness becomes near-blindness. The blind become the near-blind or, more properly speaking, the partially-sighted. And here the ray of hope still shines.

Our original question—do errors of refraction ever lead to

blindness, should now be changed to: Do errors of refraction ever lead to impaired vision or near-blindness? And another question can be added: Can refractive means ever correct near-blindness?

And the answer to both is not the unqualified no we gave before. It is yes.

When a highly myopic individual complains that his vision is failing, and spectacles do not improve the situation, he will possibly fall within our new definition.

He is suffering from progressive myopia, which becomes complicated in adult life with intraocular changes of a degenerative type. The outer layers of the eye stretch, and the inner layers—the middle choroid layer and the innermost retina, become atrophied and devoid of blood supply. This occurs particularly at the posterior pole of the eye—the very central point of vision. Incurable central blindness results, but absolute and total blindness is not the ultimate outcome. Peripheral vision remains and we have a typical situation of near-blindness.

Likewise, the person suffering from higher degrees of hyperopia often shows signs of imperfect pre-natal development and a predisposition to glaucoma because his eye is so short—his anterior chamber so shallow.

(Yet, other investigators seem to point to the intraocular pressure by elongation at the posterior pole—producing myopia. Their claim is that the young eye will yield to this increased pressure by elongation at the poterior pole—producing myopia. In the adult, where the tissues have attained greater rigidity, this elongation is not possible, and glaucoma becomes recognizable.)

In both instances it is obvious that structural abnormalities may be the common causes for progressive myopia and retinal degeneration, or for high hyperopia and glaucoma (in addition to other causes.) There is, therefore, no evidence to point to myopia of itself causing retinal degeneration, or high hyperopia causing glaucoma.

But our answer was yes because refractive errors, of and by themselves, are known to be the most important factor in another type of near-blindness—the type known as amblyopia, partial loss of vision generally found only in one eye. We have referred to this in our consideration of squint. Only in this condition does refractive defect sometimes play a great role in etiology.

In this abnormality, no organic change or disease process can be located in the eye itself. The cornea is clear, the lens unimpaired. There is no evidence of increased tension or loss of pupil reflex to light. The surface of the retina (the fundus) appears perfectly normal. There is no indication of nerve involvement or brain disturbance. From all appearances the eye and its attachments are perfectly normal, all the more credible since, in most cases, the other eye sees normally.

In some such cases (a large majority in fact) a very high degree of refractive error exists. This defect had never been corrected and it is found that even its correction at the time the amblyopia is discovered is of no avail. But after suitable training and the use of the proper correction vision is reawakened.

Theories point to an arrest of development of the macula of the eye as the reason for the amblyopia. As mentioned in our chapter on orthoptics, occluding the useful eye and stimulating vision in the amblyopic eye by suitable targets and illumination—plus the use of the proper refractive correction, frequently elicits useful vision. And in cases where a squint has resulted from this nonuse of the eye, this reawakened vision becomes an integral factor in permitting binocular fusion, frequently straightening the eyes.

It is the considered opinion of some researchers that if refractive correction had been applied sooner the amblyopia would never have developed. Whether this is so, the fact is that amblyopia is the only condition where loss or absence of vision is even remotely attributed to lack of refractive correction.

Even here, however, amblyopia may be due to some systemic cause—alcohol or tobacco poisoning, or some form of drug or focus of infection in an area such as the teeth or ears. Promptly upon removal of the cause does vision reappear.

Our second question, Can refractive means ever correct near-blindness? also received a yes answer. How do we explain this?

We have seen that modern advances have ameliorated blindness so that in effect it has become, in many cases, near-blindness, so much so that even our definition has changed. These modern advances have changed, in large measure, the complete inability to distinguish light from dark to a residual ability to see which simply awaited some method of elicitation.

Unfortunately, however, this did not alter the treatment of the near-blind person for many years. The partially-sighted individual was still taught to read and write by touch only, and in later years by recordings. When it came to occupational therapy, training was only for those pursuits where sight was not required. In these respects these unfortunates were treated no differently than the totally and irrevocably blind. For a long time no effort at all was made to utilize to any extent any remaining vision, no matter how little.

As a matter of fact, the most serious stumbling block to this utilization was the belief that it would be injurious to the eye, that it would strain the eye and result in even greater diminution of light perception. For years the partially-sighted were discouraged from employing any residual vision. From a medical standpoint—when it was determined that medical and surgical treatment could not improve the patient's visual acuity above 20/200—he was dismissed as a hopeless case. Limited vision-testing procedures used as recently as a generation ago, made it unlikely for any possible improvement of this condition.

Happily enough today this idea that a near-blind eye would be injured by use is completely discredited. The picture has changed . . . let us see how!

In probing the actual physical effects of blindness—full or partial—it became obvious that retinal changes occurred in many cases.

If opacities in the media, the cornea or the lens, or nerve or cranial involvements, were not the cause, ophthalmological diagnosis disclosed alterations in fundus appearance which were evidence of damage or atrophy. Practically all the conditions we have described have their characteristic fundus appearance which, in fact, serves as a prime diagnostic implement.

That this damage of the retinal elements was the essential

agent of vision loss seemed a warranted conclusion. Bearing this out was the fact that in cases of regeneration by medication, the fundus reassumed its normal appearance and vision was restored. (Most cases, however, are irreversible—once occurring a fundus change remains.)

In cases where only partial damage or atrophy occurred, however, it was discovered almost 200 years ago that simple magnification would be beneficial. It would serve to enlarge the retinal image so as to stimulate as many visual nerve elements as possible. The non-seeing areas of the retina would therefore be smaller in proportion to the image and interfere less with its perception. The too-few reactive cones stimulated by the unaided image would be augmented by a greater number of effective cones encompassed by the enlarged image.

While this magnification would be equally effective for distance seeing, the use of any refractive help to accomplish it was never envisioned. For near, however, many partially-sighted persons, even a century or more ago, discovered that with the use of a strong hand-magnifying lens they could continue, with bright lighting, to read. For many years no other help was available.

In more recent times these individually procured hand-magnifiers were simple convex lenses, either double or plano convex, and ranged in magnifying power from 2 to 14 times. Some came with built-in illuminators.

Not until 1948 was there even an organized effort to encourage their use. Then the American Foundation for the Blind attempted to collect various magnifying glasses, and the needy could select one best suited for their needs. (And at the same time, too, a Megascope was introduced, a projector which would throw an enlarged image 25 times the size of a printed page onto an illuminated screen. With this device some patients with a Snellen acuity of only 1% can learn to read.)

Further utilization of reading aids has led to the modern-day development of more than 200 varieties of magnifying devices. The main categories into which they fall include those worn in regular spectacle form—simply high convex lenses; those mounted

by death some who were closest to me. I do not forget them.

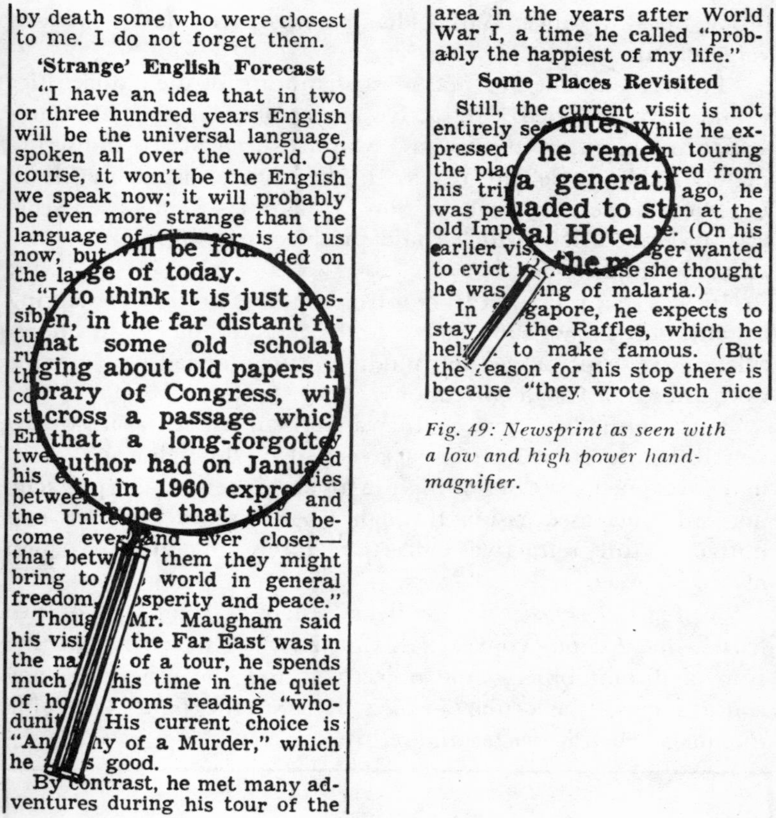

'Strange' English Forecast

"I have an idea that in two or three hundred years English will be the universal language, spoken all over the world. Of course, it won't be the English we speak now; it will probably be even more strange than the language of ꟷ ꟷ er is to us now, but ꟷ ꟷ will be foun ded on the large of today.

"I to think it is just pos sible n, in the far distant f turat some old schola ru ging about old papers i th orary of Congress, wil co cross a passage whic st that a long-forgotte En author had on Janu ed two his ties betwee h in 1960 expr and the United ope that ld be come ever and ever closer that betw them they might bring to world in general freedom, sperity and peace."

Thoug Mr. Maugham said his visi the Far East was in the na of a tour, he spends much his time in the quiet of ho rooms reading "who dunit His current choice is "An y of a Murder," which he s good.

By contrast, he met many adventures during his tour of the area in the years after World War I, a time he called "probably the happiest of my life."

Some Places Revisited

Still, the current visit is not entirely se After While he expressed he reme n touring the plac red from his tri a generati ago, he was pe aded to st in at the old Imp al Hotel e. (On his earlier vis er wanted to evict se she thought he was ng of malaria.)

In gapore, he expects to stay the Raffles, which he hel to make famous. (But the reason for his stop there is because "they wrote such nice

Fig. 49: Newsprint as seen with a low and high power hand-magnifier.

on focusable stands which can be adjusted to vary the distance from the page; and hand-magnifiers which are held by the user at a suitable distance from the reading matter.

But in all cases the limitations of the magnifying glass were extreme. First, it could be used only for reading and was of no value at all for distance viewing. Second, because of its strength (8 to 50 diopters), the field of view was extremely restricted. Oblique astigmatism and peripheral aberration were very much in evidence. And third, because of its strength, the hand-magnifier in the most practical form had to be held steady—by hand—at the proper focal distance. With older patients particularly, this was very difficult.

To overcome the first and most significant of these difficulties would have provided a refractive means of correcting blindness —restoring useful vision to those who had been placed indiscriminately in the same category as the hopelessly, incurably blind. For these neglected blind the aim of many researchers for years was to devise a lens which could produce magnification for distance viewing.

It was natural that the astronomical telescope—enlarging distant objects, would suggest itself. The simple Galilean refracting telescope proved to contain a principle readily adaptable to the needs of visual correction.

Early in the twentieth century a German scientist, Dr. Moritz von Rohr, developed a compact version of this telescope. Originally designed for cases of high myopia, his telescopic spectacles not only increased vision through magnification but also permitted a full refractive correction rarely tolerated by high myopes.

As Fig. 50 shows, the Galilean system is composed of two lenses—one a strong convex lens which focuses parallel light rays from a distant object (the objective) and the other a strong concave lens (the ocular) which diverges the light, enlarging the image when it reaches the retina.

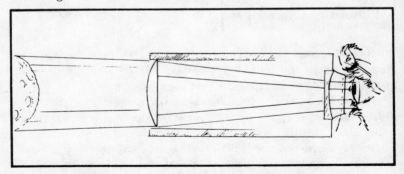

Fig. 50: The Galilean Astronomical Telescope: The objective is a strong convex lens converging the light to a concave ocular.

In adapting this to the human eye, von Rohr soon determined that magnification would be limited by one factor, the distance between the objective and ocular lenses. Mathematically speaking, magnification—while it expresses the ratio of image to object size, is determined by the ratio of focal lengths of these lenses in the system. These were necessarily very short because the focal length of the ocular must coincide with that of the objective. Magnification therefore was limited.

Figure 51B shows the resultant telescopic lens developed by von Rohr and then produced by the Zeiss optical works.

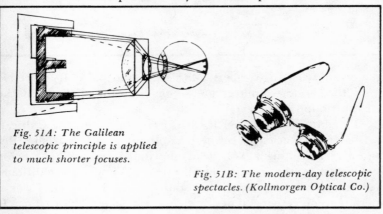

Fig. 51A: The Galilean telescopic principle is applied to much shorter focuses.

Fig. 51B: The modern-day telescopic spectacles. (Kollmorgen Optical Co.)

In its finished form the complete dimensions of the system were approximately three-quarters of an inch from front to back surface and about 2 inches in diameter. Further improvements increased the possible magnification but not without extending the front-to-back dimensions. Also, the greater magnification had the effect of narrowing the field of vision.

With the greater magnification the letter on the chart appears roughly 2.2 times the size it ordinarily is. Thus the 20/200 letter will appear as large as the 20/400 letter. For this reason, it will appear closer to the viewer.

Aside from the limited magnifying power obtainable, the Galilean telescopic system has decided advantages. It permits an erect image rather than an inverted one, and because of the

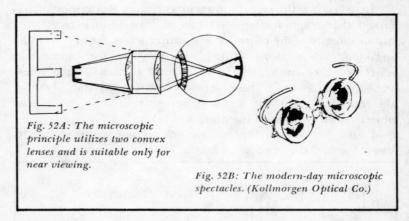

Fig. 52A: The microscopic
principle utilizes two convex
lenses and is suitable only for
near viewing.

Fig. 52B: The modern-day microscopic
spectacles. (Kollmorgen Optical Co.)

paucity of reflecting surfaces, affords a bright image. Its objective lens, furthermore, collects and condenses more light than the unaided pupil of the eye.

By adding more power in the form of a cap to the Galilean telescopic spectacle, it became possible to convert it from a distance to a reading aid. Instead of parallel rays of light being converged by the lens, as the illustration shows, the additional convex power supplied by the cap (about 8 diopters) would permit an object viewed at one-eighth of a meter (approximately 5 inches) to be magnified. This not only gained the inherent telescopic magnification of 1.8 or 2.2, but also the nearness magnification of the object being clearly visible at half the normal viewing distance (10 inches). The resultant magnification proved quite practical for reading. Additional stronger reading caps would enable even closer distances of viewing and hence even greater magnification.

A further adaptation of the telescopic system was made in the form of the "microscopic" spectacle—designed specifically for near vision. Figure 52B diagrams the effect of this lens and its resultant magnification.

With this lens both the objective and the ocular were convex lenses and the entering rays had to be divergent in order for the image to be erect. For this reason the spectacle was suitable only for seeing near objects and could provide magnification of approximately 5x.

The magnification of the 1.8 telescopic system produced as much as an 80% increase in visual improvement. However, in many cases of optic nerve atrophy and central chorioretinitis—such as produced by progressive myopia, this improvement, remarkable as it is, was not sufficient. A 2.2 telescopic system would produce 120% improvement—an increase in magnification of 50% over the 1.8.

The development of these forms of subnormal vision correction took many years. From their first appearance early in the twentieth century until the 1930s, their weight and unsightliness, plus the extreme limitation of the field of vision considerably restricted their usefulness. Little advance was made during this time.

In the decade from the 1930s to the 1940s, however, renewed interest produced improved designs which reduced weight and bulkiness. More cosmetically acceptable lenses—providing broader vision fields and greater clarity, were the product of the next ten years of research.

During the next ten years, also, greater concentration was placed on the preparation and examination of the near-blind for this type of correction. Aside from the different psychological approach necessary—the continual reassurance and essential encouragement—testing procedures were advanced radically.

Specialized Snellen charts—graduated from 20/800 to 20/70 rather than the former normal 20/200 to 20/10, were created, and a testing distance of 10 feet was used instead of the customary 20 feet. Much larger letters were used in addition to the usual smaller types.

Illumination began to play an important role. The examiner would try different lighting arrangements to arrive at the most satisfactory one for a given cause. The use of auxiliary aids, such as the pin-hole disc and multiple pin-hole disc, illustrated in Figs. 53 and 54, was undertaken more intensively in cases of media opacities.

The advantage of a pin-hole opening or openings in such

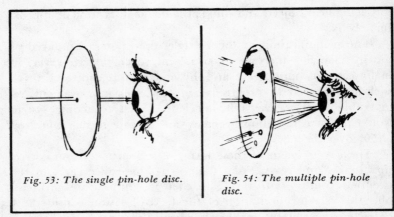

Fig. 53: The single pin-hole disc.   *Fig. 54: The multiple pin-hole disc.*

cases is that the random scattering of light by the opacities—very troublesome to the eye—is eliminated. Only narrow beams of light are permitted to enter the eye, and the pin-hole is situated in such a way as to by-pass the opacities. This limits the field considerably and cuts down tremendously the amount of light. If, however, proper illumination is cast on the object to be viewed, clear and accurate images are reproduced.

Other devices such as a stenopaic slit—which limits the entering light to a very slender slit—proved especially advantageous in cases of high irregular astigmatism. The use of special side-shields or visors to exclude oblique entering light was accelerated, as this light would be reflected by corneal and lens opacities and interfere with visual perception.

All in all, the tempo of refractive and quasi-refractive correction for the near-blind has increased immeasurably within the past decade. In many cases, although still remaining technically within the definition of "blind," partially-sighted persons corrected by these means—by telescopic, microscopic or special devices—have had new worlds opened to them.

Some who have been blind from childhood and compelled to read Braille, have been enabled to read printed books with ease. Others, blinded in adult life and forced to relinquish reading, now can resume this pastime.

Stamp collecting, photography, sewing, tooling and other crafts and hobbies became possible again for many. The resulting social and vocational rehabilitation restored many partially-sighted persons as useful, self-respecting members of the community.

Improved distance vision enabled many to enjoy television, sports, and theatrical performances—sometimes for the first time.

But most important, the telescopic, the microscopic and other special devices we have described provided new impetus to the motivation for seeing. Despite their inconveniences and limitations, they provided new avenues for research into the refractive correction of blindness . . . research which is still producing results.

And they marked the death-knell of the despairing, resigned acceptance of a fate worse than death. For they signified the end of the era of the neglected blind.

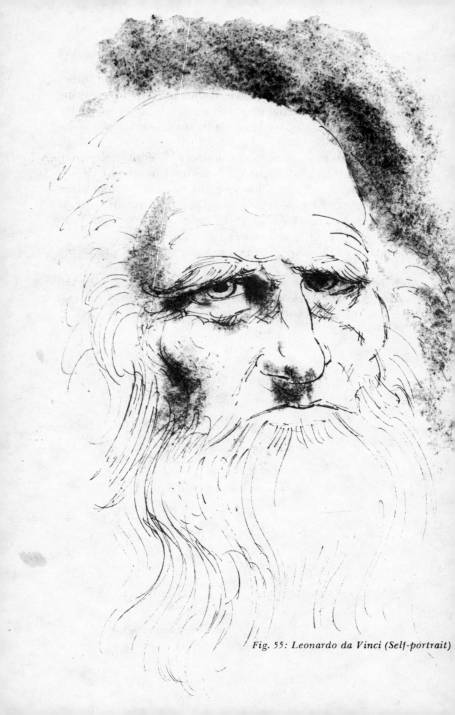

Fig. 55: Leonardo da Vinci (Self-portrait)

IX

What About Contact Lenses?

Long before any knowledge of convergence or accommodation existed, long before the precise nature of refractive error was understood, and certainly long before any theories of eye exercises or other forms of treatment were contemplated, it was obvious that objects appeared completely different when viewed under water.

To an inquiring mind it was readily apparent that light rays entering an eye under water were barely refracted. Later investigation confirmed the belief that the index of refraction of the cornea differed very little from that of water.

This indicated that if water were placed in some container in front of the eye, the corneal front surface could virtually be disregarded insofar as refraction was concerned, and light was only refracted at the point it entered the water.

That this offered a clue to replacing a defectively refracting cornea with a water lens seems to be confirmed by historical records. In the days of the Renaissance, in 1508 to be exact, we are given to understand that Leonardo da Vinci, artist, scientist and inventor extraordinaire, was able to alter visual refraction by just this means.

As Fig. 56A shows, he might have contrived to contain water in a small cup with a curved, transparent anterior surface, which could be placed in front of the eye. The water would effectively negate the corneal curvature.

Whether da Vinci conceived this because of his own purported vision loss or purely because of his speculative mind, there is little doubt that he was first to envision the possibility of placing a water lens directly on the eyeball. Quite intuitively he might have reasoned that the prime cause for visual defectiveness was the lack of proper corneal refraction and concluded that a most satisfactory correction could be obtained in this simplified fashion.

But it proved far from simple.

Many centuries passed—and spectacles and their production grew and prospered—before da Vinci's idea was carried to its next step—a thin, saucer-like glass shell which, still separated from the eye with water, fit *under* the eyelids.

Interestingly enough, however, before this stage was reached, da Vinci's observations were verified during the course of other researches. These concerned the study of luminosity of the eye—the fact that some animal eyes are lustrous and appear to glow in the dark. The cat's eye is a good example.

In 1703 the French oculist Mery found that the luminosity of the cat's eye could more easily be viewed when the animal was held under water. His explanation was that the water filled in the unevennesses of the cornea. Six years later his colleague, Dr. de la Hire, argued that the cat's fundus (back of the eye) was seen under water because of the abolition of corneal refraction. Consequently, he claimed, any light entering the eye would barely be refracted and would then be reflected by the back of the cat's eye almost as clearly as it entered.

On the same subject, one Dr. Kussmaul in 1845 actually did apply a plano-concave lens to a cat's eye to neutralize the convex power of the cornea. He hoped by this means to view the eye's interior. This attempt failed because he did not realize the necessity for illuminating the eye (a matter which Helmholtz rectified not more than five years later, leading to his invention of the ophthalmoscope) .

Almost fifty years before this, however, in 1801, Thomas Young, who described astigmatism, had rekindled the spark of da Vinci's idea. In his studies on accommodation, he was able to dismiss the cornea from consideration by finding his own accommodation unaffected when he eliminated the optical effect of the cornea. He did this by placing a weak objective lens of a microscope before his eye separated by water.

These studies verified without question the closeness of the refractive index of water and that of the cornea—they verified that new refraction would take place and usurp the function of the cornea at whatever entering surface to the water there was. They provided the basic concept of another form of eye correction.

In 1827 Sir John Herschel, the eminent English astronomer and mathematician, expressed the concept in greater detail. He suggested the use of just such a thin, saucer-like protective shell —of glass—to shield the cornea from infection due to a diseased lid. Figure 56B shows the basic nature of this device.

Likewise, Herschel proposed the use of such a shell containing transparent gelatin for the correction of irregular corneal curvature—then identified merely as astigmatism. He even suggested the utilization of gelatin-filled glass capsules to obtain an impression of the eye and then prepare accurately shaped shells from such impressions! In this, of course, he anticipated—by more than 100 years—one of the modern methods of fitting contact lenses—the molding method.

Interest in these observations could not have been acute, for sixty years elapsed before any significant progress was made.

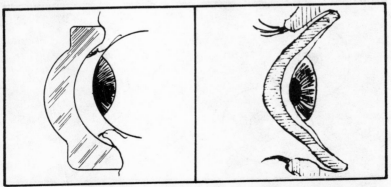

Fig. 56A: How da Vinci might have contrived to use a waterlens.

Fig. 56B: Herschel's idea of a protective shell.

During this relatively dormant period advances in optics and physiology confirmed the following basically sound conclusions involved in the ideas of da Vinci, Young and Herschel:

—that the index of refraction of the cornea was close to that of water (1.39 as compared to 1.33) and not too far from that of glass (1.49).

—that the cornea was the major refracting surface of the eye.

—that the white part of the eye—the sclera—was relatively insensitive to touch or pain.

—that the cornea had a physiological need for natural moisture supplied by various secretions.

With the climate of ophthalmology what it was sixty years after Herschel, advance crowding advance, it is not surprising that some daring steps were finally taken.

In 1887 an important first took place. A thin, transparent glass shell was blown (much glass was blown in those days) and designed to fit beneath the eyelids and rest directly on the white sclera of the eye.

The shell was made at the request of a German physician, Dr. Saemisch. It was similar to an artificial eye except that it had a transparent central portion instead of one painted to match the normal eye. Artificial glass eyes, used to this day, were known even during the Middle Ages. They were merely colored glass—

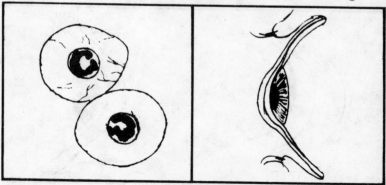

Fig. 57A: The resemblance of the shell to an artificial eye was marked.

Fig. 57B: It fit under the lid completely clearing the cornea.

shaped to fit the socket of a missing eye. Dr. Saemisch simply wanted a thin shell to fit over his patient's eye (still with useful vision) in order to protect it from a diseased lid—the very protective idea proposed by Herschel!

An expert glass blower succeeded in making such a shell. The patient wore it quite satisfactorily, and it served its purpose well until his death some twenty years later.

But even at the same time this cosmetic or prosthetic shell was being fabricated and worn, a noted Swiss physician, Dr. A. E. Fick, was conducting experiments with fully transparent eyeshells on rabbits and cadavers purely for refractive purposes.

These experiments marked the birth of the "kontakt brille," or contact lens, the name these transparent shells bear to this day.

Dr. Fick did not succeed in these experiments, despite the cooperation of the famed Zeiss optical works. But the results of his research formed the basis for eventual success.

Two years later, in 1889, the first successful contact lens ground to a refractive prescription was created, and the fact firmly proven that, optically, vision could be corrected by such a lens. Working closely with a Berlin optician, a young medical student, August Muller, designed a lens to correct his own extreme nearsightedness.

Despite attempts with many, many lenses of different shapes and sizes, Muller was unable to get a properly fitting one and he eventually abandoned the idea. But not before he proved conclusively that his nearsightedness could be corrected equally as well with a contact lens as with regular glasses.

Figure 58 shows such a lens with the ground-out central portion containing the prescription. It is almost a spherical lens yet is basically similar to the almond-shaped lenses of future years.

This was the first step in replacing the front corneal surface. By making the new surface more curved than the cornea itself, more refracting power would be provided. By making it less curved, it would lessen the refractive power.

As Fig. 59 shows, the equivalent effect of a concave—a divergent or minus spectacle lens is produced when the front surface of the contact lens is less curved than the corneal surface.

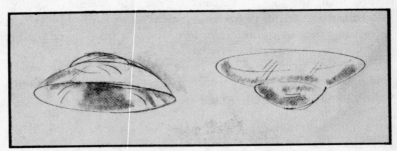

Fig. 58: All-glass contact lenses as made by Zeiss.

For the nearsighted eye this lens will serve to lessen the refraction at the front surface and therefore bring rays to a focus on the retina.

Similarly, Fig. 60 shows the effect of a contact lens with a front surface more curved than the corneal surface.

The equivalent effect of a convex—a convergent or plus spectacle lens is created, serving to increase the refraction of the eye and therefore shorten the focus of the rays so they fall on the retina. The farsighted eye is thus corrected.

The groundwork was laid by August Muller. That his idea was entirely practical as well as theoretically sound was definitely proven from an optical standpoint. Later discoveries emphasized the wondrous nature of the contact lens as a refractive device.

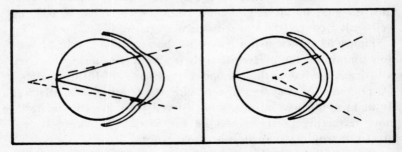

Fig. 59: The concave contact lens has a flatter outside curve than the corneal surface.

Fig. 60: The convex contact lens has a steeper outside curve.

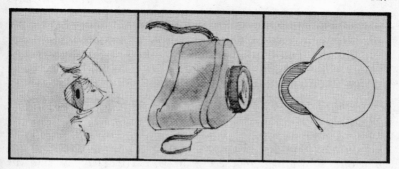

Fig. 61: In keratoconus the cornea assumes a bulging, cone-like curve.

Fig. 61A: The "hydrodiascope"—no more than a water lens in front of the eye.

Fig. 62: The contact lens provides a new front surface to keratoconus.

And, of course, they also revealed the magnitude of the fitting problem.

History records the next major advance in 1912, when the Zeiss optical works produced contact lenses, still made of glass, for use in keratoconus, the obscure condition causing the front surface of the cornea to bulge into an irregular, cone-like shape (Fig. 61).

Keratoconus had long been known as a condition not correctable by ordinary glasses (despite the abortive attempt of Sir Christopher Wren to utilize hyperbolic glasses). Because of the lack of the essential element of a geometrically perfect optical surface to the cornea this condition remains uncorrectable by regular glasses.

The earliest method for improving the vision in these cases was by the use of a water-cup strapped to the eye above the brow, the so-called hydrodiascope (Fig. 61A). The water equalized the irregular curve of the cornea and the convex lens in front replaced the power of the cornea. In a way, this resembled da Vinci's original idea.

But the contact lenses produced by Zeiss seemed to provide the answer—an entirely new surface which would negate the corneal distortion.

Figure 62 shows the corneal deformation of this condition and how it is neutralized by the contact lens.

This was hailed as a major ophthalmological advance and contact lenses became the treatment of choice for keratoconus. Greater acceptance was to follow.

It was shortly after this that the study of glaucoma—the dread cause of blindness we have already discussed, received important impetus through the medium of a contact lens. Researches to this time had verified glaucoma as due in part to improper circulation and drainage of the eye fluids, particularly through the aqueous which occupied the eye's anterior chamber. Methods of investigating this drainage which permeated the so-called anterior angle of the chamber—the angle formed by the back surface of the cornea where it joins the sclera and the ciliary body which supports the iris, were handicapped because of the difficulty of viewing this angle.

In 1914 Dr. Maximilian Salzmann, an Austrian ophthalmologist, utilized a contact lens to found the study of gonioscopy, the viewing of this anterior angle. Until then it was virtually impossible, even with ophthalmoscopy and the slit lamp, to see any but the deepest anterior angles. As Fig. 63 shows, a ray of light coming from the anterior angle would generally be reflected so that it did not reach the observer's eye.

With a contact lens we have seen that a new front surface to the cornea is provided. The effect is invariably to deepen the chamber. As Fig. 63A shows, any ray then is permitted to emerge and open the angle to view.

With this extremely important application of a contact lens, Dr. Salzmann helped immeasurably in the diagnosis of the course and treatment of glaucoma. Further advances—adapting prisms and mirrors in front of the contact lens to facilitate observation, have made gonioscopy a vital tool in glaucoma research.

It is interesting to note that before Dr. Salzmann used a contact lens in this manner, other physicians had filled the patient's lower lid with water and instructed the patient to look down so that the cornea was immersed in the water. In effect this provided a new surface to the cornea and thus deepened the cham-

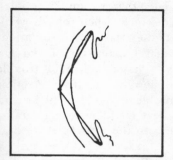

Fig. 63: Light rays from the normal anterior angle are reflected by the corneal surface interiorly.

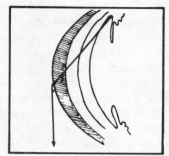

Fig. 63A: By deepening the anterior chamber with a contact lens, the same light rays are then refracted outside the eye to the observer.

ber. Viewing of the anterior angle could then be done after a fashion. A fortuitous adaptation of da Vinci's fundamental theory of applying a water lens to the eye!

Also in 1914 Zeiss and the Mueller optical works produced lenses for use in cases of post-operative cataract (aphakia) to compensate for the loss of the crystalline lens of the eye. The considerable plus power required was successfully ground onto the front surface of the contact lens and these patients too were accepted as worthy subjects for the still-experimental lenses.

Not until 1929, however, barely a generation ago, did the application and use of contact lenses for irregular astigmatism—a condition allied to keratoconus in its distortive effect on the cornea, become known.

Until this time, it must be remembered, the utility of contact lenses was limited to individuals who were virtually sightless and who were not amenable to correction by ordinary glasses. August Muller's original application of contact lenses for near-sightedness was rarely employed; and would-be wearers endured the oft-protracted discomfort and even pain frequently involved in fitting and wearing lenses of that era. The almost magical improvement in vision offered by the lenses made the trials and tribulations well worthwhile.

It was not realized until much later that a complex problem of corneal metabolism was involved which, when solved, would eliminate the pain, the discomfort, the trials and tribulations. It took many years to determine that impairment of tear and air circulation to the cornea was a major source of trouble, that interference with the natural flow of nutritive secretions through the cornea was a serious problem, and that disturbance of the eye's capacity to dissipate heat could not be tolerated. These were the true stumbling blocks to the wearing of a device directly in contact with the eye.

The lenses then in use were virtually all the large type illustrated in Fig. 58—resting directly on the white portion of the eye. The arched, central portion cleared the cornea and was generally filled with a so-called neutral or "buffer" solution, such as bicarbonate of soda or boric acid to which the eye ostensibly did not react.

Experimentation continued with other designs none the less, some of them much smaller. In point of fact, even the modern-day corneal type lens—the lens whch floats only over the central corneal section and has no contact whatsoever with the white of the eye, was anticipated by a German physician years before 1929. Because of poor optical quality and excessive thickness of the lens, however, the idea was never followed through.

Likewise, experimentation continued with different buffer solutions of varying concentration to simulate more closely normal tear secretion. But progress could not be hurried.

Thus, practically all contact lenses were the large, scleral type. Zeiss ground lenses and Mueller blown lenses were dominant. Their usefulness at this time was still considerably limited because accurate measurement of the eye was not yet possible. Even the molding method of fitting had not yet been devised, and Zeiss and Mueller lenses were so-called stock lenses—produced at random and in large quantities so they might be used in trial and error fittings.

In 1932 came a major breakthrough. A prominent Hungarian physician, Dr. Joseph Dallos, experimented and succeeded in using a special molding plaster to secure an accurate cast of the living eye. This meant that the shape of the scleral section of the lens could be virtually a replica of the sclera of the eye. It provided a theoretically perfect-fitting lens.

Such a lens was still filled with the same buffer solution used in the earlier lenses. Any attempt to eliminate this would cause a large air bubble to appear in the central section which still cleared the cornea. The result would be blurred vision. Otherwise, the molded lens fit snugly on all contours of the white of the eye.

Whether a lens with such a glove-like fit could be worn remained to be proven. Disappointingly, only a very moderate degree of success was attained. Wearers found that despite the greater comfort of the fit, vision became blurred after a few hours, just as it had with the older lenses.

They found the eye began to burn or feel warm. They complained that a "tight" feeling developed, as though the lens were a tight bandage. Evidently, circulation of some sort seemed to be impaired, even more so than with trial and error lenses.

In addition, wearers discovered that when the lens was removed it was completely dry—no buffer solution remained.

These difficulties led to the conclusion that the solution was absorbed by the corneal tissue. Examination immediately upon removal of the lens confirmed the presence of corneal swelling, substantiating the tightness so frequently reported. Distortion was evident in the shape of the cornea, so much so that after removal of the lenses, hours later in many cases, vision was blurred even with ordinary glasses.

Only limited improvement, therefore, could be credited to molded lenses. Variations in the size of the corneal portion of the lens—attempting to permit greater freedom to the cornea, made little difference. Even a return to preformed lenses and trial-and-error fitting, embodying some newer processes and techniques, was still unproductive.

Meanwhile, during the mid-1930s, plastic—a substitute for glass—developed to the point where it could be ground with equal precision and accuracy. Methylmethacrylate, the same plastic used in plexi-glass and lucite, was found to be ideal for optical purposes and, equally as important, completely non-reactive to the eye and its secretions.

With contact lenses, moreover, the shape of the finished product could, if made of plastic, be altered by heating and grinding—an impossibility with glass. Even greater accuracy in conforming to the shape of the eye and fitting the lens to its irregularities could be attained.

But plastic provided no answer to the basic problem of achieving sustained wearing time with comfort and without after-effect.

A new approach involving the use of molded (and pre-formed) lenses without fluid was attempted. The objective: somehow to permit the tears and secretions of the eye to per-meate under the lens and thereby keep the cornea moist. Prior tests had proven conclusively that a dry cornea soon lost its transparency and protracted dryness might result in permanent damage.

The mid-1940s brought the design of molded fluidless lenses with channels and perforations in the scleral section. In this manner, tears were permitted to flow through to the cornea. These tears collected in the precorneal space sufficiently so as to prevent the air bubble which would have appeared had the older-type lenses been applied without fluid. Figures 64A and 64B show these modifications to the molded scleral lens.

Similarly, preformed scleral lenses were adapted for use without any foreign fluid by fitting the outer rims so that they extended away from the sclera, allowing space for tears to enter (Fig. 64C).

Nevertheless, full success was still beyond realization. Sur-prisingly enough, however, these fluidless scleral lenses gave results as good or better than those with fluid. Wearing time and comfort, in many cases, were greatly improved. The annoyance of a foreign fluid and its marked corneal after-effect was elim-inated. Yet constriction and tightness around the cornea still seemed to develop and extended wearing time for most wearers was not a practical reality.

Thus the search continued.

Finally, in the late 1940s, in the course of continuing experi-

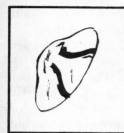 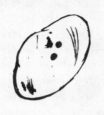 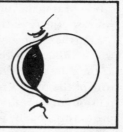

Fig. 64A: Two channels generally extended from the bottom of the lens to the corneal section.

Fig. 64B: Perforations, sometimes one, two or more, were made directly below the corneal section.

Fig. 64C: Without channels or perforations the lens might be fit so that its edges stood away markedly.

ments, the cycle reverted to the lens formerly attempted and discarded . . . the lens which fit only over the cornea and had no scleral section. Now made of plastic, this newly-named corneal lens was thin, light, and of good optical quality. It showed great promise.

It was a tiny, spherical disc, slightly smaller than a dime, approximately ½ inch in diameter and 1/50 inch in thickness. The prescription was ground onto the outer surface as in all previous lenses, and the inner surface was designed to touch the cornea only at its center. Just as the preformed scleral fluidless lens did, the rim of the lens stood away in order to allow tear and air passage.

It was a lens which could not possibly produce any constriction around the cornea . . . it required no fluid at all . . . and could conceivably solve the problem. It became the precursor of the modern-day contact lens.

This was another bold forward step—for the very thought of placing a lens directly on the most sensitive part of the eye was repugnant to orthodox ophthalmological teaching. Yet it did not take long to deduce that this sensitivity of the cornea was aroused only by minute sources of irritation on highly localized areas. Any gross pressure sensation did not produce pain or irritation.

If you close your eyes and then press—through the lid and directly onto the cornea—you will feel no pain, simply the sensation of touch. And should you touch the cornea without closing your eye the sensation will be the same—touch, but no pain.

Further, the belief, formerly universal, that no contact lens would adhere to the eye without anchorage under the eyelids—as the scleral lens had, was shown to be false. The natural moisture of the cornea provided enough capillary attraction or surface tension to permit the lens to adhere quite strongly. You can prove this, too, by simply moistening your fingertip and touching it to a small piece of tissue paper one or two inches square. The paper will cling to your fingertip.

Figures 65A and 65B show this primitive type of corneal lens and also how it adhered to the eye.

Practically speaking, the corneal lens was nonirritating to the corneal surface because of the relatively wide area it covered. Indeed, it could hardly be felt, and adherence of the lens to the cornea was excellent.

But two serious flaws soon became apparent.

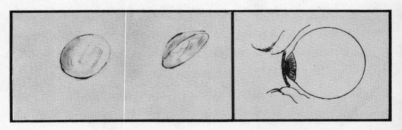

Fig. 65A: The original corneal lens.

Fig. 65B: Its edges stood away to permit entrance of tears.

You will notice in Fig. 65B that the edge of the corneal lens stands away from the corneal surface. This was a must. How else could tear and air and necessary secretion flow to keep the center of the cornea moist? The eyelids—never a problem with scleral-fitting lenses, now posed a serious obstacle.

Because the edge of the lens stood away from the cornea, the lids felt the foreign object in the eye. This feeling, in many cases, was highly irritating—sufficiently so as to make the wearing of the lens, comfortable if the lids were held apart, quite unbearable if they were free to blink normally.

At the same time this blinking of the lids was often sufficient to move the lens out of place—to occasionally dislodge it completely—even though it stayed in place perfectly with the eye wide open.

By the nature of its fit, too, the central part of the corneal lens came in direct contact with the cornea, as the illustration shows. Frequently this not only prevented proper moistening of the cornea, but also caused, on occasion, some peeling of the cornea's outer tissue layer. The results were temporary loss of transparency of the cornea and what is known as an "abrasion" —the actual rubbing off of corneal tissue. The latter condition required a sustained nonwearing period for regeneration.

For these two reasons, therefore, lid sensation and effect on the cornea, the newly-developed corneal lens fell short of satisfaction. Further improvements of the corneal lens—aiming to reduce its size, its weight and its thickness as well as improving its optical qualities, did nothing to resolve these problems. But it became increasingly apparent that if these two problems—and these two problems alone, could be solved, a genuinely successful contact lens was at hand.

And a successful contact lens would accomplish many things:
—The benefits of refractive correction would be enhanced.
—The lens would eliminate the restriction of the visual field which glasses necessitate.
—Reflections from glasses would be obviated.
—The aberration and distortion effect—particularly when objects are viewed obliquely through high prescription glasses, would be eliminated.
—Rain or snow, heat or cold would offer no hazards.
—Image size because of prescription strength would not diminish or enlarge—thus allowing two entirely different eyes to work together.
—Pathological and physiological conditions not correctable by glasses would be corrected.

And in addition to all of these, the lens would be practically invisible when worn.

The stage was set, the problems clearly seen, and the goal within reaching distance.

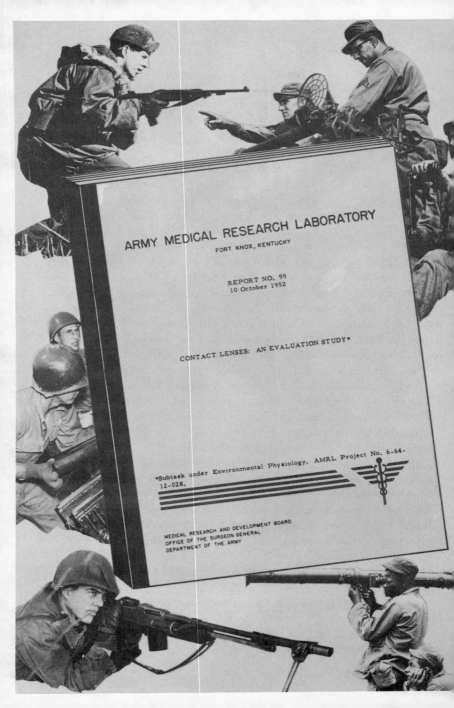

ARMY MEDICAL RESEARCH LABORATORY

FORT KNOX, KENTUCKY

REPORT NO. 99
10 October 1952

CONTACT LENSES: AN EVALUATION STUDY*

*Subtask under Environmental Physiology, AMRL Project No. 6-64-12-028.

MEDICAL RESEARCH AND DEVELOPMENT BOARD
OFFICE OF THE SURGEON GENERAL
DEPARTMENT OF THE ARMY

X

The Army Fights
Eye Problems

It was at this pivotal point in the development of contact lenses that important impetus was given to sight-without-glasses research.

The Army undertook a full-scale project to examine a problem of enormous magnitude—the eyeglass-wearing soldier. In October, 1952, its report titled "Contact Lenses: An Evaluation Study," was issued.

The introduction to the report stated the following:

"The object of this project was to make a comparative study of four types of contact lenses and spectacles to determine the relative merit of each and thence to ascertain the feasibility of using them for selected members of the Armed Forces.

"The potential advantages of contact lenses to military personnel would appear to be numerous if such lenses proved practical. The possible utilization by the Armed Forces of large numbers of men previously disqualified or on a limited duty status served as one reason for undertaking this study. Furthermore, men who ordinarily wear eyeglasses could perform better in inclement weather and participate in field duties previously considered impractical. The danger of lost, broken, or fogged spectacles might be eliminated. Light reflections from spectacles which may reveal positions to the enemy could be eradicated. The problem of using spectacles with sighting equipment as well as the use of inserts in gas masks might well be simplified. Contact lenses themselves offer numerous advantages in increasing the visual field, elimination of corneal astigmatism, etc.

"Among the disadvantages to be considered would be the expense, fitting and adaptation time, the development of corneal haze and the resultant subjective fogging of vision and chromatic halo, variable tolerance and photophobia, ocular irritation, etc. However, in view of recent advances in design and manufacture, the potentialities of contact lenses deemed a study such as this advisable."

Based on the rejection rates in World War II and the Korean conflict, the percentage of disqualifications because of poor eyesight was inordinately high. Limited duty assignments given because of visual defects were also alarming.

Aside from this, it was quite obvious to the Army that the eyeglass-wearing combat soldier was actually a menace. His glasses could fog up at critical times; they could be blurred by rain, snow, sand or mud. The bespectacled soldier could be a danger to the men beside him as well as to himself. His glasses might shatter in training; they might break in a combat area where replacement glasses were not accessible. He could be injured more severely in accidents because he wore glasses.

On the desert his glasses could become spotted with perspiration; in the Arctic they would frost over. He could adapt very slowly—if at all—to a sudden need for new confining headgear, or to the use of sighting devices, in situations where adaptation could mean the difference between life and death.

Military
Disadvantages
of
Eye Glasses

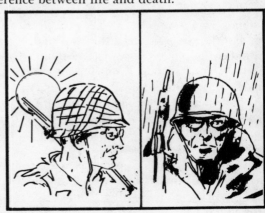

Certainly, he would be seriously handicapped if plunged into a predicament where swimming was essential. In the field— where he might be subjected to jolting, jarring, and similar circumstances, glasses might prove a fatal drawback.

And, of course, his own need to wear glasses and the fear of possible resultant mishaps might very well becloud the soldier's ability to think clearly and react quickly.

An episode during the course of the Army's tests clearly illustrated the point. One contact lens wearer, required to crawl through a barbed wire entanglement, was struck in the eye by a barb. His eye was saved only because the cornea was protected by the lens. The best he could have hoped for had he been wearing spectacles was that the glasses would merely have been broken, leaving him without visual correction at a critical point.

In another instance a contact lens wearer was accidentally struck in the eye with a belt buckle. His eye was uninjured. With glasses he would not have fared better than the aforementioned bespectacled soldier.

In both cases the contact lenses were a decided advantage, not only maintaining visual acuity at a crucial time but actually protecting the eye from possible serious injury.

For a long time the Armed Forces were acutely concerned with these problems. The Army Medical Corps had studied various techniques of sight correction, such as drug therapy and

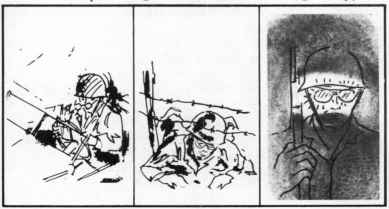

eye exercises. Results were relatively inconclusive and unsatis-
factory.

It was quite natural, therefore, to turn to the newest form of
vision correction—contact lenses. In its study, the Army used
two lines of inquiry.

First, the practicality of contact lenses—their application,
wearing and after-effect, was compared with ordinary eyeglasses.

Second, four types of contact lenses were tested and compared:

1. The plastic scleral lens using artifically supplied fluid
(sodium bicarbonate solution) .

2. The plastic scleral lens channelled to permit the wearer's
natural tears to circulate. The channel extended upward from
the lower center of the lens to the corneal section (Fig. 64A) .

3. A fluidless glass lens with a small circular hole about 1mm.
in diameter just below the corneal area, again to permit free
circulation of the wearer's tears (Fig. 64B) .

4. The corneal plastic lens, the one recently reintroduced
(Fig. 65A) .

Throughout, the Army referred to the fluidless scleral lens as
ventilated lenses.

The fitting time for each of these lenses varied considerably.
Two hours and fifty-five minutes were needed for the corneal
lens, three hours and thirty-three minutes for the fluid scleral
lens, eight hours and forty-five minutes for the fluidless plastic
scleral lens, and nineteen hours for the fluidless glass lens.

In all cases all the lenses were fitted to each individual in a
selected group of volunteers who had diversified visual defects.
In addition, all were fitted with spectacles.

After fitting was completed, a program of testing was established to cover both field and laboratory work. Attempts were
made to duplicate most of the possible situations encountered
by a military man in routine army life and on the field of battle.

The volunteers joined with basic training units for exercises
necessitating acute vision, physical strain, and exposure to the
elements. They performed such exercises as tank driving (day

and night), rifle and machine-gun firing, infiltration, and hand-to-hand combat.

Performance was checked while the troops wore gas masks, stood guard duty . . . even when on kitchen police. To observe the effect of the jolt of an opening parachute, training towers were used. Field and obstacle running, and swimming conditions were reproduced.

Spectacle and contact lens wearers were tested under temperature extremes of —40° and +120° Fahrenheit in hot and cold laboratory rooms. The effects of an altitude of twenty thousand feet was simulated in the low pressure chambers of Wright-Patterson Air Force Base. The effects of explosive decompression also were observed.

Photophobia, light tolerance and dark adaptation were charted. Visual acuity, depth perception and color vision were tested. Binocular vision and fusion, muscular balance and reflexes were checked. The effect of radiation on plastic versus glass lenses and spectacles was determined. The overall protection of the eye by the lens covering was investigated. The effect of perspiration, the practicality while swimming, even the psychological state of the eyeglass and contact lens wearer, were explored.

In short, the first thorough and exhaustive study by a government agency in the field of spectacles and contact lenses was conducted.

It brought forth a wealth of fruitful results and had far-reaching effects, indicating that contact lenses possessed inherent and indisputable advantages over spectacles—they offered more protection, afforded better vision, and in practically all other particulars overcame the disadvantages of eyeglasses. In the words of the report:

"In field requirements, where the individual may undergo extreme physical activity, jolting, jarring, and exposure to varied material obstacles, spectacles are at a disadvantage because of their vulnerable position. They are easily dislodged and broken. Contact lenses not only temper these problems, they also offer further protection to the eye. They also reduce the mental con-

Contact Lenses Found Useful for Troops

By the Associated Press.

CHICAGO, Oct. 14—Contact lenses—thin glass or plastic shells worn on the eyeballs—have many advantages for troops, eye doctors were told yesterday.

The general conclusion of a report on recent tests by the Army Medical Research Laboratory was that contact lenses were superior to spectacles on sports or battle fields.

Dr. James L. McGraw of Syracuse and Dr. Jay M. Enoch of Fort Knox reported:

"Rain, snow and mud, which may interfere with vision when spectacles are worn, are not problems with contact lenses. The frosting and steaming of spectacles is avoided with contact lenses."

Also, "spectacles are at a disadvantage" because they are "easily dislodged and broken."

"Reflections from spectacles may reveal a hidden position to the enemy, this is not so with contact lenses. Contact lenses may protect the eyes from foreign bodies and direct trauma (injury). They also offer varying degrees of protection against harmful radiation."

The report was made at the annual meeting of the American Academy of Ophthalmology and Otolaryngology, a society of eye, ear, nose and throat specialists.

Article from New York World-Telegram and Sun, October 14, 1953.

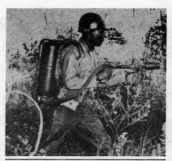
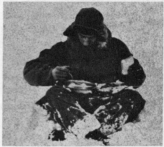
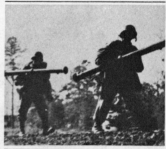
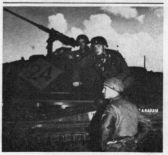

cern that the spectacle wearer naturally exhibits in the face of physical obstacles.

"The protection that contact lenses offer to the eye cannot be overlooked. Not only do they protect against foreign bodies and direct trauma, they also offer varying degrees of protection against radiation.

"The visual limitations that spectacle frames create and the aberrations existing in high power lenses are eliminated when contact lenses are employed."

On the other side of the coin, certain disadvantages of contact lenses were brought out:

"The most outstanding disadvantages of contact lenses at the present time are the cost, time, and the skill required for fitting."

Easy loss of the lens because of its size is mentioned; also cited is the high motivation needed for the individual to be fitted. Essentially, however, these were practical problems well realized before 1952 and were still to be solved.

But the report went further. In analyzing the reactions of wearers of each of the four types of contact lenses, it produced highly significant findings.

The study verified the belief that corneal metabolism was impaired by the fluid scleral lens. Progressive corneal clouding and swelling resulted from absorption of the sodium bicarbonate solution. Hazy or fogged vision occurred. A scattering of colors by the swollen tissues caused a colored halo to form around lights. A marked diminution in visual acuity and an increase in light-irritability occurred. Increased time was needed for dark adaptation, and, most important of all, extended wearing time was unattainable. After approximately three hours of wear, visual acuity began to fail and the cornea became progressively cloudier.

With the fluidless scleral lenses reactions were greatly improved. Even after six hours there was little decrease in visual acuity, and at no time was there any measurable halo effect. Without doubt this indicated an absence of corneal swelling or absorption. Nevertheless, wearing time was still less than hoped for (approximately six to eight hours) because of lens constriction surrounding the cornea. This clogged the free passage of tears and air.

With the corneal lens, also, there was little reduction in visual acuity, and there could have been greatly extended wear with no halo effect. But only with the corneal lens were the serious drawbacks of lid irritation, easy dislodgment, and corneal abrasion evident. Nearly all participants in the project complained of these conditions. Several experienced considerable discomfort to the point where the lenses were intolerable. Because these factors limited wearing time, they were as serious as corneal swelling and clouding, if not more so. Photophobia, too, appeared more pronounced with corneal lenses, but this was ascribed to mechanical irritation and poor tolerance.

Basically, the Army's study confirmed the findings of previous investigators that the chief requirements of a wearable contact lens were:

- Proper tear and air circulation to the cornea.
- Unimpaired movement of nutritive fluids through the corneal tissues.
- The maintenance of the eye's capacity to dissipate heat.

The research offered a comprehensive and independent appraisal of the lenses then in use and, in step-by-step analyses, pointed out findings with each. And then it drew its conclusions.

The study demonstrated that the most satisfactory contact lens of all was the ventilated fluidless scleral lens. In a lens of this construction "neither glass nor plastic was deemed better for fabrication" but the plastic lens "offers greater protection to the eye."

Most important, there was no doubt that "the vented fluidless corneal-scleral lens that permitted a free flow of tear fluid and aeration of the cornea was superior to other designs."

The report mentioned the greater simplicity in fitting the corneal lens as compared with the scleral lens—under three hours necessary for the corneal lens, almost nineteen with the scleral. It referred also to the far easier procedure involved in applying corneal lenses to the eye as contrasted with the scleral lenses.

But the most significant conclusion was unquestionably contained in the fact that the ventilated fluidless scleral lens was found to be the most comfortable, and the corneal lens to give the longest wearing time—when it could be tolerated.

The scleral lens—fitting snugly and ventilated to be fluidless, caused no lid or corneal irritation, yet did not permit sufficient wearing time because of eventual constriction around the cornea.

The corneal lens—because it had no scleral section and did not constrict the cornea, permitted excellent wearing time. Yet it was uncomfortable because loose fitting—necessary for normal tear flow, led to lid and corneal irritation.

Both lenses were fluidless, both depended on proper circulation of tears and air beneath them. Four to eight hours of comfortable wear with the scleral lens was achieved; eight to twelve hours and longer wear with the corneal lens, when it could be tolerated.

Contact lens fitting was on the horns of a dilemma.

The next avenue of research, however, was clearly indicated. The comfort of the scleral lens and the wearing time of the corneal lens must in some way be combined. If this could be accomplished, the realization of a centuries-old dream and the achievement of a whole new means of refractive correction was in sight.

And, surely enough, this was the avenue where success was found—thanks to the Army Medical Report No. 99.

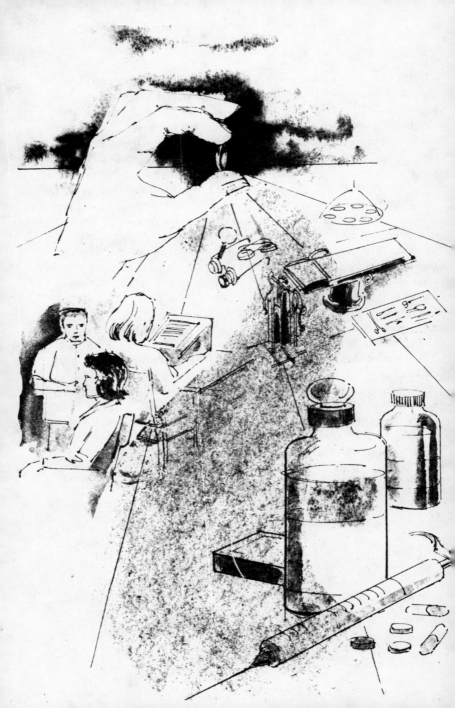

XI

The Way Is Pointed

It was only a matter of months before a theoretical concept of a lens combining the advantages of the ventilated scleral and the corneal lenses evolved. In early 1953 the answer was proposed —a corneal lens properly ventilated with an edge that did not stand away from the cornea.

A simple solution—a ventilated corneal lens—yet one which required years of experiment and trial before it could be utilized in finished form. That form was the vented lens.

This was a lens which fit so that its edge did not stand away from the cornea and the center section did not rest on the cornea. It possessed four tiny grooves, or vents, around the inside of the rim, permitting the passage of tears and air beneath it.

An original article in the professional press which heralded the introduction of this lens declared, in part:

> . . . a lens had to be devised which was tight enough to permit adhesion under all circumstances, and yet which had properties permitting the normal metabolism of the cornea to be unimpaired . . .
>
> "The vented, grooved lens is the product of patient research and trial with various notchings, perforations and islands. It maintains minimal thickness (between .15 and .20mm. throughout) and has, at four equidistant points along the inside perimeter, four precisely ground-out semi-circular grooves. These grooves are approximately 3mm. in diameter and extend to within 3½mm. of the apex, thus

permitting a pupillary aperture of 7 to 8mm. These grooves
reduce edge thickness by approximately .05mm. . . .

The vented lens allowed the free flow of tears and air by
refining all the advantages of the corneal lens—reducing weight
to less than 1/750th of an ounce, diameter to approximately
1/3rd of an inch, and thickness to less than 1/100th of an inch.
The four grooves around the edge led directly to the center, and
between the grooves the edge followed the shape of the eye
perfectly—without standing away. Thus, lid sensation, irritation
and dislodgment were substantially eliminated.

Not to be overlooked was the fact that this vented corneal
lens in effect created an air space between its center and the
front surface of the cornea. Thus, the risk of an abrasion—ever-
present with a corneal lens in direct contact with the center of
the cornea, was practically non-existent.

The advantages of the lens were manifold. Gone was the risk
of dislodgment. Gone too was the likelihood of the lens drifting
off center.

New vistas in fitting accuracy opened.

Formerly, the corneal lens and even the ventilated scleral
lens had to be fit loosely, and therefore approximately, to permit
adequate tear flow. Now, a lens could be fit precisely to the
corneal contour. The entire art of contact lens fitting was on the
road to becoming an exact science rather than a trial-and-error
experiment.

The new vented corneal lens proved to require fewer adjustments, fewer wearer visits, than any prior lens. Approximately
two-thirds of the formerly needed fitting time was eliminated,
and a basic reappraisal of the whole theory of contact lens fitting
was in order.

Now the natural inclination of ophthalmological opinion to
allow a desirable area of clearance between the central section
of the cornea and the inner surface of the lens could be followed.
In this area—narrow though it was, natural tears could collect,
form a fluid lens and fill in any irregularities in the corneal
curve. The movements of the eyelids, moreover, were found to
aid the circulation of tears and air within the grooves into this

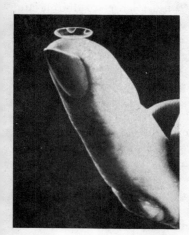

Fig. 71A: The vented lens.
(Vent-Air Contact Lens
Laboratories)

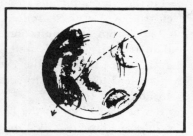

Fig. 71B: The vented areas
permit passage of tears and
air. (Following arrow).

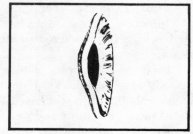

Fig. 71C: The lens is shaped to
follow the eye's curve.

central space. Corneal nutrition and transparency was un-impaired; the sensitive apex of the cornea was untouched.

In a very real sense, the vented lens came to dominate the contact lens picture. It became evident, as a result of thousands of pairs successfully fittted, that practically speaking contact lenses had arrived.

Yet one problem persisted. Apparently minor, it became more nagging as fitting techniques improved. This was the hydrophobic property of the poly-methyl-methacrylate plastic used since 1936. It caused dryness of the lens' outer surface. Here moisture was essential in order to permit smooth lid movement. Now it reasserted itself as other problems subsided. The so-called "wetting agents" to overcome it were moderately effective, but research continued to look for a better answer.

Further developments to adapt contact lenses to double and even triple-vision needs followed within a short time.

Aside from the limitations of ordinary glasses, the bifocal and/or trifocal wearer is well aware of the additional handicaps they impose. Training the eye to move from one part of the eyeglass lens to another in order to utilize the different focuses, is troublesome to many.

If you try to look at the floor through the reading section of the bifocal glass, it will appear very blurred and much closer than it actually is. Walking up or down stairs, for this reason, can be somewhat hazardous—particularly to older people whose reflexes are slow to respond to danger.

In driving a car, where perfect distance vision is so essential, the bifocal section may interfere with the view of the dashboard, or block the view when a sudden nearby side view becomes imperative.

Even modern forms of bifocal eyeglass lenses only partially remedy these drawbacks. Judgment of an object's positioning is improved, but distortion is still present; the reduced section—deliberately minimized so as not to interfere with distance, presents a problem when reading. The head must be held in a more or less fixed position. In many instances therefore the angle of reading or working is very awkward.

The bifocal wearer who changed to contact lenses simplified his problem a great deal. He could wear his lenses for distance vision and when reading or working at close range would simply slip on a pair of regular glasses containing the additional magnifying power necessary. Actually his situation was that of an individual who did not need glasses at all for distance and was merely presbyopic (needing accommodative help for near vision).

Indeed, the fact that few bifocal wearers became contact lens wearers until the advent of the vented lens, was because all-day wear was not a practicality with distance contact lenses. It was not because they objected to wearing an auxiliary pair of glasses for near vision. This was always preferable to bifocals. With the vented lens assuring comfortable wear, bifocal wearers became anxious for the benefits of the single vision contact lens.

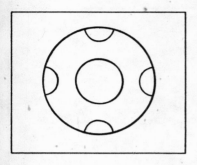

Fig. 72: The bifocal lens showing the ring for near vision.

Research efforts to modify the contact lens to permit the bifocal spectacle wearer to enjoy near vision proceded apace. Grinding the lens with two sections—an upper and lower, simulating the regular eyeglass bifocal, proved fruitless, because the contact lens of itself might rotate out of position. Attempts to keep the lens in a stationary position were dismissed as impractical.

Finally, in 1958, researchers came up with a workable solution —two distinct circles of vision. The central circle—about 1/5 of an inch—would continue as the portion devoted to distance vision and would be completely rimmed by a circular band— 1/8th of an inch wide—ground to the near prescription.

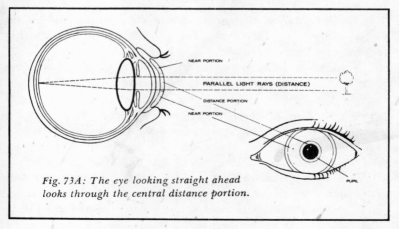

Fig. 73A: The eye looking straight ahead looks through the central distance portion.

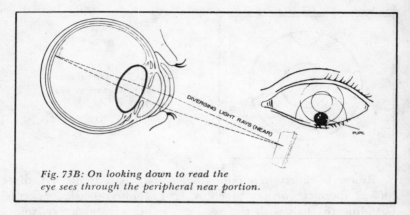

*Fig. 73B: On looking down to read the
eye sees through the peripheral near portion.*

The lens was designed to move upward slightly when the
eye's gaze was downward. This was caused by a combination
of factors. First, the eye muscles and the corneal tissue of the
upper part of the eye would tense and retain the lens as the
eye turned downward, and second, there would be a slight
upward pressure of the lower lid on the lens as the eye turned
under the lid.

Both factors combined to bring the near band directly into
the line of vision. When the wearer looked directly ahead, the
lens would resume its normal position.

The mechanics of fitting this new bifocal vented lens required
extreme care and accuracy . . . a far cry from the primitive fitting
methods used only a few years before.

In addition, isolated experimental cases of trifocal wearers
were fitted, and in these instances a second circular band was
employed and ground to a prescription intermediate in strength
between the distance and near power. It served to permit the
wearer to view objects at a working distance—approximately 25
to 40 inches, in addition to the near distance of 10 to 25 inches.

It appeared that with the vented lens in single vision, double
vision, and triple vision form, all the benefits of contact lenses
could now be offered eyeglass wearers, almost irrespective of
refractive correction. It remained only for the practitioner fitting

lenses to undo the harm and the fear and the ignorance which older, non-successful lenses had induced.

For this, a coherent, scientific fitting procedure had to be followed. For this, the effects of wearing the new lenses had to be thoroughly determined—their pros and cons exhaustively investigated, documented and revealed, so that the stage could properly be set for a true evaluation of the new vented contact lens in the field of visual correction.

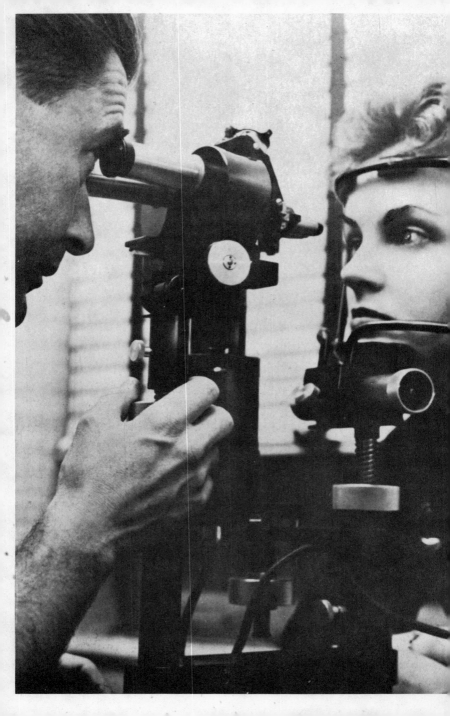

XII

How Are Contact Lenses Fitted?

There is a parallel readily apparent between spectacle and contact lens fitting in their early days. As we have seen, spectacle fitting by trial-and-error was the rule until the mid-nineteenth century. It might easily be said that trial-and-error contact lens fitting was the rule until the mid-twentieth century.

Years ago, would-be contact lens wearers were required to sit patiently while one lens after another was tried and discarded—a technique based purely on the fitter's conjecture as to the required lens.

Later on (and even today), a semi-liquid plaster was poured into a perforated shell and applied directly onto the eye. Even with anaesthesia—only sometimes employed, this procedure was highly uncomfortable and troublesome. Moreover, the anaesthetic did not prevent eye movements, making the process quite inaccurate.

This plaster formed a mold while in contact with the eye which was then used as the female for a positive cast. The cast served as the basis for preparing the contact lens, which was formed to fit this shape perfectly. Over the central corneal section of the cast there was a "buildup" of additional material to create a space between the lens and the cornea. In addition, this central section was ground out so that about 1/25th of an inch was the closest the lens came to the cornea.

When artificial fluid was used this space sometimes increased 1/12th of an inch; without artificial fluid the space was narrowed, for it was filled only with tear fluid.

In all cases, whether artificial fluid or natural tears were involved, the outer curvature of the finished lens' corneal section was the factor which determined the prescription. The inside curvature was more or less constant, but the outside curve was made steeper or flatter depending on prescription requirements— plus or minus.

The contact lens—once it was returned from the laboratory, would then be applied to the patient's eye. If a pre-formed or so-called trial lens were used—from sets of these lenses which manufacturers distributed—such a lens would be applied.

Checking and correcting the vision of the wearer through the contact lens would follow. In subsequent visits, the physical fit of the lens would be checked—tight or loose areas of the scleral section were determined and adjusted, and any manifest constriction of the cornea or pressure at its apex was uncovered. Attempts were made to eliminate these faults.

Finally, instruction in the application and removal of the lenses was given. With the artificially-supplied fluid, there was the problem of retaining enough solution so that an air bubble did not appear. Repeated attempts were sometimes necessary to accomplish this. Then there was the use of a suction cup to remove the lens. Lids would tighten involuntarily and the wearer would blink his eyes when the suction cup approached. Only great perseverance would finally enable the patient to overcome this reaction.

At last he was ready to wear the lenses. In cases where the artificial fluid was used, it was generally a $1\frac{1}{2}\%$ solution of sodium bicarbonate—sometimes supplied by the fitter, sometimes secured in a pharmacy, but most often prepared by the wearer himself. The wearer had to guard against impurities in the solution. Only double-distilled water, not available everywhere, had to be used; it had to be discarded and renewed frequently.

The schedule of wearing time was a rigid one. For the first week the lens would be worn for $\frac{1}{2}$ to 1 hour intervals, two or three times per day; for the second week, 1 to 2 hour intervals, two or three times per day, and so on until maximum wearing time was achieved. Unfortunately, this maximum rarely exceeded three to five hours.

When the fluidless scleral lens was employed, the nuisance of applying the solution-filled lens was eliminated. Still the application procedure was cumbersome. These were the necessary steps:

- The upper lid had to be held high.
- The lens had to be slid well up into the eye chamber.
- The lens was covered by the upper lid which was held tightly in place over it.
- Then the lower lid was tugged gently out from under the lens.

With the fluid lens, the wearer had to bend over so as not to spill the fluid; with the fluidless, he could slip the lens on while his head was upright. But aside from this, the bulkiness of each lens necessitated much the same steps.

Wearing time with the fluidless lens started also with $\frac{1}{2}$ to 1 hour periods, two or three times per day. But it kept increasing until, not infrequently, six to eight hours, and occasionally longer wearing time was reached.

The wearer usually made repeated visits to the fitter's office so that the various symptoms which developed after several hours of wear could be diagnosed, and attempts made to correct difficulties. The ultimate success, as we have mentioned before, was limited.

But in fitting both scleral lens types the only basic shape involved was the contour of the sclera—since the lens rested there and completely cleared the cornea. Because the scleral surface is irregular and incapable of measurement, either the molding technique or the trial-and-error technique was used to arrive at a lens which appeared to approximate its shape.

Observation of the appearance of the sclera with the lens applied—to note any blanching or constriction of scleral blood vessels or actual pressure on the scleral tissue, was the only way of judging a correct scleral fit. The ideal lens, obviously, was one which seemed to follow the scleral contour very closely, and was neither too loose nor too tight.

Corneal measurements in scleral lenses were unnecessary except as a possible aid in determining the prescription. This was superfluous, however, because the use of a finished scleral lens which fit the eye approximately could easily be used as a basis for the needed prescription. Here the lens already had a prescription in it, and any change necessary to achieve proper vision could be ground either onto the same lens or a more accurately fitting one.

With a corneal lens, however, fitting procedures changed radically. Molding and large, preformed trial lenses were unnecessary. The sclera became completely divorced from the fitting and measurement of the cornea became paramount. The width of the cornea—its height and, most important, its curvature, had to be accurately measured and provided for.

Furthermore, the eyelids—with which contact lens fitting heretofore had not concerned itself, became increasingly important. The palpebral opening (the space between the upper and lower lids while the eye is normally open) and the tightness or looseness of the lid tissue itself proved to be significant factors in tolerating the corneal lens—particularly the early ones.

In fitting, this space between the lids and the lid-tightness would, in large measure, determine the overall size of the lens. And these were complicating factors. The degree of tightness would often vary—depending on the particular stage of the fitting and the wearer's psychological state. Many lids gave the appearance of tightness in the initial fitting stage and relaxed later on, necessitating a change in fitting. Also loose lids might tighten up later and present a problem to the fitter as well as the wearer.

Fortunately, with the vented lenses these factors were virtually eliminated.

So that how a contact lens is fitted today is entirely different from the way it was ten years ago. In addition to the regular eye-testing procedure to determine the defect of refraction—the same eye test you undergo for ordinary glasses—the fitting of the modern-day vented corneal lens follows a highly precise pattern.

The approximations of scleral lens fitting are past and the early efforts of corneal lens fitting have been superseded. These early corneal lenses were fit with the inside curvatures flatter than the corneal curve; the center portions, as previously described, touched the apex of the eye's cornea, and the edges stood away from the eye. Figure 65B shows this.

The modern vented lens, however, by its nature, must be fit precisely to follow the shape of the cornea so that the edge does not stand away. Figure 71C shows this. The need for this essential precision led to a reevaluation of the instruments used in contact lens fitting.

The eye-testing instruments we have already described—the ophthalmoscope, the ophthalmometer, the retinoscope, the trial frame and lenses (the phoropter)—these are the basic essentials of any refracting test.

With corneal contact lens fitting the ophthalmometer (or keratometer, literally, "cornea-measurer") assumed far greater importance than in either spectacle or scleral lens fitting. This instrument—by the effect of reflection, enables the observer to determine the actual curvature of the cornea's front surface. It becomes the key instrument in the fitting of all corneal lenses.

Physiological studies over many years had determined, however, that the corneal curve is not a spherical one—in fact it resembles a parabolic curve with only the very central section a true sphere. This section is a 4 to 5 mm. (1/6th to 1/5th of an

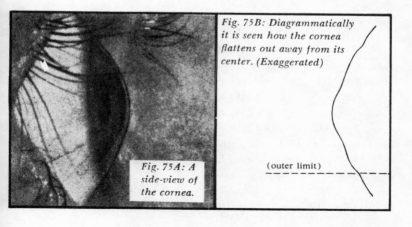

Fig. 75A: A side-view of the cornea.

Fig. 75B: Diagrammatically it is seen how the cornea flattens out away from its center. (Exaggerated)

(outer limit)

inch) circular area immediately around the optical axis of the cornea. Outside this area, as Fig. 75B shows, the curvature diverges sharply from a spherical form—flattening out to become, in many cases, quite astigmatic and irregular.

This fact was of little consequence with the corneal lenses since only the center actually touched the cornea. With the vented lens, however, it became very significant. Here the edges did not stand away and had to be fit to this outside corneal curve.

A limitation of the ophthalmometer then became quickly apparent. Essentially a reflecting device from a spherical surface, the ophthalmometer could not be utilized to measure this peripheral parabolic surface. As a matter of fact, no optical device heretofore devised could measure this surface—if indeed it could be measured at all by optical means.

The vented lens thus brought with it a serious handicap to be overcome. Its very accuracy demanded a more complete and more accurate measurement of the cornea—from it apex to its outermost periphery.

This problem was approached by the creation of an instrument called the corneascope (Fig. 76). It was a photomicrographic device which, by accurate focusing and enlargement, gave a photographic, measurable record of the shape of the eye in one of the most important dimensions for contact lens fitting—the vertical dimension.

Invented in 1958, the corneascope was planned to fill the void left by the limitations of the ophthalmometer and provide accurate means of fitting the vented corneal lens. An exact replica of the eye's curvature could be used in fitting the lens precisely to the corneal surface.

As is commonly the case with scientific advances, the corneascope had still another valuable function. Because of a photometric attachment it was able to determine the intensity of light reflected from the cornea. As a camera, it would record this intensity.

The value of this lay in the fact that the intensity of reflected light is directly affected by the transparency of the cornea. Thus,

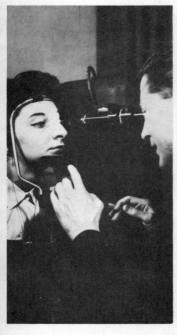

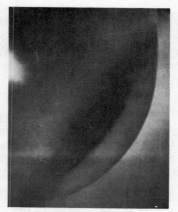

Fig. 77: A magnified corneascopic photograph (Contact Lens Specialists)

Fig. 76: The "Corneascope." (Contact Lens Specialists)

any loss of transparency immediately shows up as a loss of reflectivity. And a loss of transparency (affecting visual acuity) has been known for a long time to be the effect of an improperly fitting contact lens. Proper corneal nourishment and metabolism being impaired, the clouding of vision and resulting turbidity of the cornea immediately show themselves in this loss of transparency.

Indissolubly linked, this transparency and reflectivity could easily be ascertained by a ray of light cast onto and reflected by the cornea. A record of the intensity of this ray could be retained by the corneascope—at the inception of lens wear, during the course of wear, and upon removal. Changes in reflectivity could then be pin-pointed and a fitting cause determined and hopefully solved.

This was a very valuable application indeed for it provided a scientific, objective appraisal of the effect of improperly seated lenses and over-wear. This precise form of reflectivity eliminated the dependence on the wearer's own statements regarding blur, fogging or cloudiness. The corneascope's photographic record of the vertical corneal dimension, it turned out, could not be precisely measured as an accurate measuring device could not be found. And its limitation to the profile reading was a continuing drawback. Its use of frontal photography, however, provided the impetus for later instruments to measure the corneal surface and complement the keratometer.

Another instrument, formerly in routine use in eye examinations, also became increasingly important in proper contact lens fitting. The slit lamp (Fig. 78), casts a highly concentrated slit or beam of light on the corneal surface and the various layers of the cornea. It penetrates to reveal the depth and structure of the anterior chamber, the crystalline lens, etc. It served in routine examination to highlight opacities or any abnormalities in tissue structure.

With contact lenses, the slit lamp revealed changes in tissue structure or any congested or bruised areas. It revealed any haziness or swelling of the tissue cells. With the vented corneal lens it could even trace the passage of tears or tiny air bubbles under high magnification. Any interruption of flow over the cornea could be detected.

In addition, a vegetable dye known as fluorescein is used. This harmless dye was introduced in 1938 and has kept pace with the progression of contact lenses in their various stages. It was added to the artificially-supplied fluid in the fluid-type lenses or placed within the fluidless scleral lenses in order to color the fluid or tears—making them visible to the observer.

Viewed under so-called "black" or ultra-violet light, fluorescein caused the fluid behind the lens to fluoresce—to emit a greenish-yellow light. It illuminated the areas occupied by fluid and therefore revealed where excessive contact was present.

With corneal lenses it would show exactly where the lens touched and if and where the lens was tight or loose. Further, any part of the cornea which had been bruised or abraded by

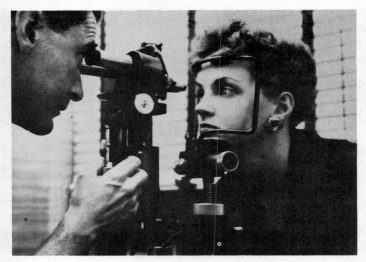

Fig. 78: *The Slit-lamp in use. (Contact Lens Specialists)*

Fig. 79: *Sections of the eye viewed by the slit-lamp.*

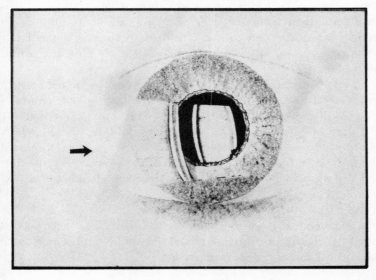

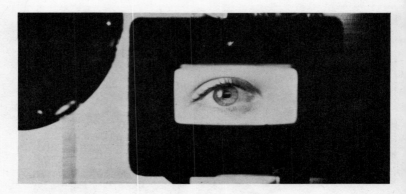

Fig. 80: The eye as viewed through the "black-light" lamp.

improper application or by malfitting would absorb some of
the dye and emit a greenish glow.

For these reasons fluorescein assumed even greater importance
in the fitting of corneal lenses—particularly the vented lenses.
It showed how tears and air flowed under the lenses; it pinpointed any abrasions. Under high-power magnification, as it is
commonly used (Fig. 80), or with the slit-lamp, fluorescein
enables the modern-day contact lens fitter to uncover immediately
any sparsity of natural circulation or an early clue to corneal
tissue change.

A very welcome result also of the success of the vented corneal
lens was that the vexatious problem of application and removal—
long so difficult and dreaded by the scleral lens wearer—became
a matter of great simplicity. No fluid could be spilled which
would produce an air bubble and which would require repeated
attempts at application. No excessive maneuvering of the lids
and sliding of a large lens deep into the eye chamber was necessary.

As Figures 81A, 81B, and 81C show, simply separating the
lids and bending over the lens was sufficient. The lens needed
merely to be clean and moist, and it would almost pop onto
the corneal surface of its own accord.

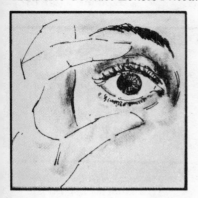

Fig. 81A: *The lids are separated.*

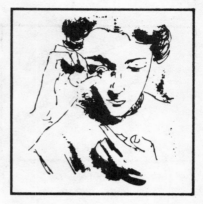

Fig. 81B: *The lens is held on the forefinger . . .*

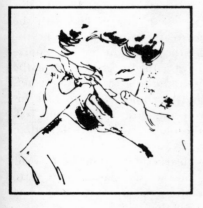

Fig. 81C: *. . . and applied directly to the cornea.*

Similarly, the problem of removal of the lens—formerly a matter of considerable dexterity and requiring the unpleasant application of the suction cup to the lens—was remarkably simplified. Merely pressing the lower lid beneath the edge of the lens and giving it a slight tug outward was sufficient to remove the corneal lens. Figures 82A and 82B show the ease of this process.

Most gratifying of all, however, was the accelerated wearing schedule the new wearer was instructed to follow. Before receiv-

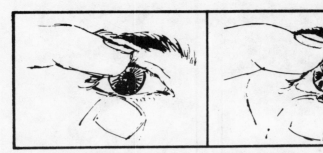

Fig. 82A: *The lower lid is*   Fig. 82B: *. . . and the upper*
pulled tautly outward . . .   *lid gently presses the lens out.*

ing his lenses (usually at the last fitting visit), he would in most cases wear his lenses as long as six to eight hours. During this time the objective fit of the lenses would be checked with the methods we have described. The wearer would be taught the proper application and removal procedures during the course of this wearing. And he would have gained a good deal of the confidence and reassurance most important to a new wearer. He would be ready—physically and psychologically, to take his new lenses with him—a far cry from the path of doubt and lack of confidence many wearers of the older lenses were forced to follow.

The new vented lens wearer's instructions would be to wear them for 2 to 3 hour intervals for the first day or two; 3 to 4 hour intervals for two days thereafter, and increase his wearing time by about one hour per day after that.

Perhaps after two or three weeks he would return for a check-up. Usually no adjustment would be necessary, but if so, it would be a simple one. In the preponderance of cases, it would be one merely to correct excessive tightness or looseness. And the procedure for correcting either condition has been so well codified that, very likely, the adjustment would require only a few minutes. Wearing would barely be interrupted.

More and more a similarity of contact lens fitting with the highly advanced fitting of modern dentistry is approached—an anticipated, prescribed mode of procedure having its basis in full knowledge of the physiological processes involved.

In brief, this is the step-by-step story of the fitting of the modern-day vented corneal lens:

Following ordinary eye measurement, the instruments and techniques we have described reduce contact lens fitting to a most simple series of tests and check-ups. By comparison with older fitting methods, the experience is an infinitely more pleasant one. Certainly it is a far cry from the trials and tribulations undergone by the wearer of years ago. The molding and trial-and-error methods are gone, the fear and dread of lenses being repeatedly applied and removed dissipated. Not more than four or five visits would generally be necessary.

Wherein then lie the disadvantages of today's vented lenses?

What, if any, is their effect on the eye?

And how far along the road to improved refractive correction will this lens take us?

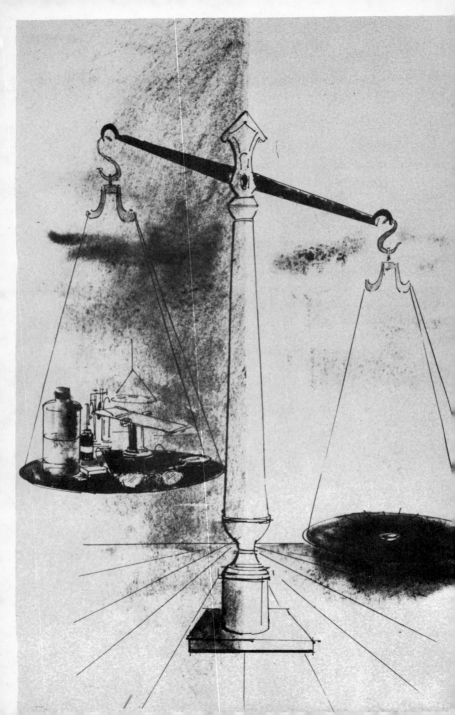

XIII

The Modern Vented Lens—Its Pros and Cons

Years before the Army Medical Report, the effect of contact lenses while being worn and their after-effect was the subject of investigation.

Precisely what corneal change took place?

What visual phenomena resulted?

What persisted after contact lens wear?

To what extent did this depend on the accuracy with which the lens fitted?

How much was inherent in the nature of having an object in such close proximity and contact with the eye?

And what would be the long-term effect?

The Army report did much to answer these questions, but these facts were already known:

With the fluid lens and again with the fluidless scleral lens, absorption of the imprisoned fluid—whether artificial or natural, occurred and corneal swelling resulted. Loss of transparency of the cornea and clouding of vision became evident.

Objective inspections of the cornea by means of the retinoscope and the ophthalmometer disclosed distortion of the corneal surface. To the wearer, vision was blurred by a haze and a colored halo appeared around points of light. In practically all such cases, the swelling subsided upon lens removal and the cornea quickly resumed its original shape. The haze and colored halos disappeared and vision was returned to normal with regular spectacles.

Even when the fluid or fluidless scleral lens was worn over a period of years, this effect resulted, but it never failed to disappear after lens removal.

In many cases of fairly habitual wear of scleral lenses there seemed to be a loss of sensitivity of the cornea. A thread, for instance, touched lightly to the cornea uncovered by the lens, failed to elicit the quick blinking reflex normally present.

Again, this sensitivity returned after a period of abstinence from wearing the lens. It seemed purely a transistory and not-too-consequential effect. Yet it was there, and lingering doubts as to its effects remained in the mind of the eye practitioner. Perhaps this was one more reason why the scleral contact lens never quite received full professional acceptance.

With the corneal lens, however, the problem of absorption was eliminated. Fluid could not collect under the lens long enough to be absorbed. But, because the central section of the corneal lens rested directly on the apex of the cornea, there was that sloughing off of surface tissue previously discussed. And there was the direct central contact—frequently pressing in the corneal surface and producing distortion which remained even after the lens was removed.

There were two effects sometimes resultant upon this.

First, there was the removal of part of the outer protective layer of the cornea, the outer epithelium—the cornea's chief guardian against infection. The abraded area became more exposed to bacterial infection, but fortunately the nature of the tissue is such that it regenerates very quickly—even when the immediate damage appears to be very severe. With ordinary cleanliness and the avoidance of any other irritation the abrasion would generally heal in a matter of hours, sometimes without the wearer even being aware of it.

Second, there sometimes appeared to be drying of the outer layer, because the free flow of fluids in and out of the tissue was prevented by the lens contact. Again, this would be relatively slight, because removal of the corneal lens for just a short period would serve to regenerate the tissue.

In both cases, corneal lens wearers would notice haziness of vision and a decrease in visual acuity after removal of the lens.

The persistence of this haziness and vision loss varied with the amount of interference with normal metabolism present—sometimes minutes, sometimes hours, and even days or weeks. With the absence of any other complicating factors, the corneal tissue would invariably return to normal and lens wearing was resumed. In no cases was any permanent effect noticed.

Concomitant with these effects a loss of corneal sensitivity was noted, similar to that experienced with scleral lenses. Interfering with corneal metabolism at the apex of the cornea—the central area primarily essential for sight—caused this. The rich supply of nerve endings in the center (richer than in any other part of the cornea) was deprived of proper nutrition, hence their excitability diminished. Removal of the cause here too—by not wearing the lenses, soon restored the sensitivity.

But unquestionably this tissue abrasion, central corneal pressure and loss of sensitivity were significant deterrents to the more widespread application of the corneal lens not only for cosmetic purposes but for severe visual problems.

There was also the factor of lid sensation caused by friction with the edge of the corneal lens. However, this was a highly localized irritation—much as a speck in the eye, and disappeared promptly when the lens was removed. Any inflammation of the inner surface of the eyelid, generally the upper, would subside immediately.

With the vented corneal lens, however, these troublesome problems were solved. Because no fluid collected under the lens, there was no corneal swelling. Because its center did not touch the apex of the cornea, there was no corneal pressure or flattening which dried the central area. Because its vents permitted an uninterrupted flow of normal tears and air over the entire surface of the cornea and especially the apex, nerve sensitivity was not impaired by the lens. And because its edge did not stand away from the cornea, there was no lid friction and irritation.

In addition, experiments indicate that the cornea can and does utilize oxygen directly from the air as part of its normal metabolism. This is all the more reason why an uninterrupted flow must be allowed. Neither the scleral lens nor the corneal lens permitted this.

The vented lens did.

None of the effects of swelling, pressure, constriction or lid sensation manifested themselves during the fitting, the wearing or after the removal of the vented lens. Visual symptoms indicative of an interruption in corneal metabolism—haziness, cloudiness, halos—were absent.

Close examination with the ophthalmometer, the retinoscope, the corneascope, the slit-lamp and the special black-light magnifying-lamp, revealed no change at all in the corneal surface. It vindicated the belief that any difficulties were due entirely to an interference with corneal metabolism and that a contact lens, of and by itself, would not cause any untoward effect—provided it did not impair normal nutrition and tear circulation.

Studies, however, did not end here. They brought to light another effect—an effect which somehow did change the total refraction of the eye in a most desirable way.

When it came to myopic wearers, the effect of the lens apparently reduced the myopia in many cases. And in other myopic cases it retarded its progression. An unlooked-for result, yet one not entirely unsuspected.

For several years, many contact lens wearers and fitters had noticed that changes in prescription, particularly for nearsightedness, seemed remarkably infrequent when contact lenses were worn. Improvement in vision—not only when lenses were first worn but consistently thereafter, seemed disproportionate to the theoretical optical correction. In a way the gain seemed to resemble the sometimes-surprising benefit resulting from visual training or eye exercise.

Why?

A number of theories were put forward.

Some ascribed the improvement in vision to the psychological lift which resulted from discarding eyeglasses . . . from the freedom of vision enjoyed and the relaxation of tension which led to strain and resulted in further vision impairment. There is a great deal of merit in this, for, as we have seen, the psychosomatic cause of a visual defect is indeed a deep-seated one.

Others ascribed it to the enlarged field of vision afforded by

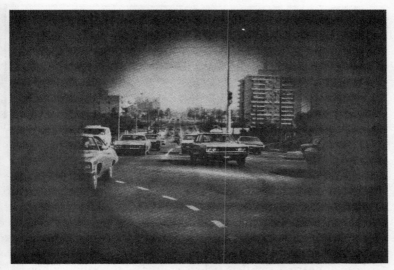

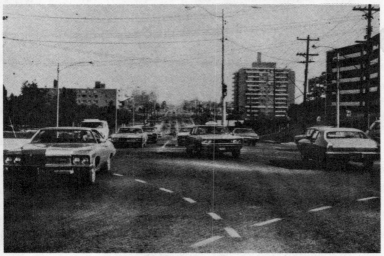

Fig. 83: The upper photograph is the constricted view seen by a post-cataract patient. (It might as well be that seen by a highly-nearsighted one.) The lower view is that seen by the same patient wearing . . . contact lenses. (Photo courtesy of B. J. Slatt, M.D., and H. A. Stein, M.D.)

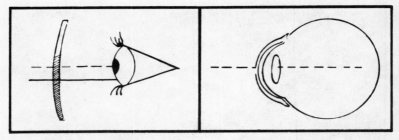

Fig. 84A: The optical axis of
the eyeglass does not necessarily
coincide with that of the eye.

Fig. 84B: The optical axis of
the contact lens becomes one
with the eye's.

the contact lens. Visual awareness increased, a heightened sense of security in one's surroundings resulted, and a lessening of tension ensued.

Others felt that the more normal image size seen with contact lenses especially by the near-sighted person made sight easier. Objects appearing smaller (when viewed with ordinary glasses) than they actually were and causing even greater eyestrain, appeared their normal size when viewed with lenses. Strain, therefore, would be reduced.

Another vein credited the better vision resulting from contact lenses—leading to the decreased need for prescription change—to the greater homogeneity of the eye's refracting system with a contact lens. With ordinary glasses there would actually be two optical systems, frequently with lines of vision at angles to each other. (Fig. 84A and 84C.) With a contact lens in front of the eye, the lens would be fit so that its optical line of vision coincided with that of the eye and turned with the eye. (Fig. 84B and 84D.)

There is no doubt that with the vented lens eliminating the extraneous factor of interrupted metabolism, a more optically satisfactory corrective means had been achieved. The benefits to the nearsighted—particularly the progressively-increasing nearsighted—were very real.

Controlled studies with hundreds of myopic cases bore testimony to this. In virtually all cases there was no increase in myopia while lenses were worn, and in a goodly number of cases

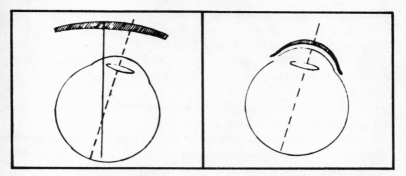

Fig. 84C: Particularly on turning the eye's optical axis separates from the eyeglass' axis.

Fig. 84D: But even on turning both the contact lens' and the eye's axis coincide.

myopia was actually reduced. If the nearsighted person put aside his lenses and resumed wearing his regular glasses, the original eyeglass prescription proved too strong. If he continued wearing his glasses, his eye would shortly revert to the former state of greater nearsightedness.

Yet, close corneal examination after removal of lenses usually revealed no change in corneal curvature which might cause this— no distortion, flattening, or swelling. Therefore, the effect could not be ascribed to a physical alteration of corneal shape—reducing its refracting power—due to the contact lens. Evidently, it was purely a psychological phenomenon affecting visual acuity.

What this meant to the thousands of parents of nearsighted children, and what it will mean to future parents and their myopic offspring, can only be conjectured. It does appear, however, that a much more effective means of myopia control has been achieved with the vented lens—a restraint and arresting of myopia more palatable and more simply utilized than other, more doubtful means such as bifocals, prisms or ocular exercises.

The same studies we have cited also bear out the stabilizing influence exerted by a contact lens over other refractive errors. Very likely the same reasons persist: better imagery, lessened psychological tension, better centration of the optical system, better fusion of both eyes, and greater clarity and field of vision.

Whether the eye is farsighted, nearsighted or astigmatic, the contact lens becomes the most effective and important single element in its complete optical system, replacing the cornea and therefore usurping more than 3/4ths the refractive power of the eye. Its function and effect is entirely different from the purely accessory effect on the eye's optical system induced by a spectacle eyeglass.

So it is not surprising to expect startling results from the wearing of these almost invisible lenses.

Their use became greater for purely prosthetic purposes—to restore normal appearance to an eye disfigured or discolored due to pathological processes. The lens would be colored to match the normal eye and both eyes would be perfectly mated.

The use of highly-tinted vented lenses in cases of albinism—an abnormal deficiency of pigment in the iris layer, became more practical. The lenses successfully filtered the entering light and relieved the extremely painful sensitivity to light generally present. Ordinary tinted eyeglasses—unless they completely shielded the eyes, could not do this. Besides, they made the wearer conspicuously handicapped. With contact lenses the eyes were restored to a more normal appearance and the wearer could less self-consciously participate in his social environment.

Frequently, remarkable improvements visually as well as psychologically resulted.

One significant case dealt with a nine year old albino child who had been in a sight-conservation class, and was also regarded as mentally retarded. His refractive condition showed a high hyperopia, but most important he could hardly hold his eyes open because of the extreme light sensitivity. His school work was far below average and his life outside school highly restricted. Typically albino, he was an extremely fair, reddish-haired child.

The change produced by substituting colored yet practically invisible contact lenses for his inadequate glasses was truly remarkable. His eyes opened in more ways than one.

Rather than avoid any direct gaze, he would look right at the person speaking to him. His personality changed overnight. Instead of barely being a follower, he became a leader, for his vision had been bettered too. He no longer had to attend a sight-conservation class and, far from being considered retarded, his school work improved to such a degree he was among the top students in his class.

Sufferers from aniridia (complete absence of an iris) found the new wearable lens a heaven-sent boon. In such cases, a virtually opaque lens—with a minute central opening (2 to 3 mm. in diameter) acting as a pupil, provided an ideal substitute for the missing iris.

What other advantages or disadvantages did this new method of vision correction possess?

We have already mentioned the utilization of contact lenses in cases where ordinary eyeglasses did not correct vision—in keratoconus, aphakia or corneal irregularity. In corneal scarring —the result of many eye diseases, a profile cross-section under the microscope reveals sharp peaks and valleys. Using a contact lens, as Fig. 85 shows, the hills and valleys are filled with tear fluid and therefore a new front surface and media become effectual.

Vision is frequently improved in such instances from an indeterminable low to close to 20/20. A useful application of this is in cases of corneal grafting. Often the corneal graft develops folds or irregularities well compensated for by a contact lens.

The new contact lens proved valuable in another area. They seemed to ameliorate to some degree the condition known as aniseikonia—a difference in image size between the two eyes. Unknown interior causes create such differences sometimes approaching 5 to 10%. Eye fatigue and discomfort, headaches, and inability to concentrate result because the eyes cannot adjust to more than a 2 or 3% difference.

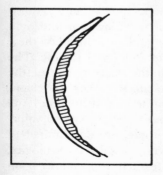

Fig. 85: The contact lens provides a new surface and media to the irregular cornea.

It was found that the wearing of one or two contact lenses served to reduce this image size difference. Specially-designed spectacles to correct aniseikonia—spectacles which were expensive and intricate—frequently became unnecessary.

Furthermore, cases of migraine headaches—that troublesome condition whose cause has eluded science for countless years, have been found in certain instances attributable to aniseikonia and amenable to correction by contact lenses. Even an occasional case of squint which is not due to hyperopia and is uncorrected by ordinary glasses would seem to respond and be reduced by the application of contact lenses.

With the achievement of satisfactory wear of the vented lens more advanced uses for contact lenses beckoned.

Many other instances of what we have called subnormal vision and described in our chapter on the near-blind became more suited for remedy by this new form of refractive correction.

In some of these, the use of the same principle as the aniridic lens proved beneficial. A pin-hole opening in the lens— just like a pin-hole disc, could be placed in such a way as to direct entering rays of light away from opacities in the cornea or crystalline lens. The same effect as the pin-hole or multiple pin-hole disc could be created. Restoration of useful vision in these cases was even greater than with the regular pin-hole disc, since occlusion of the opacities of the eye was so much more effective with the opaque contact lens.

A further use became practical—also in the cases of the near-blind.

The telescopic and microscopic spectacles had many shortcomings. Aside from the limitations of magnification and field of view, and their obvious weightiness and unsightliness, these spectacles demanded almost complete immobility of the eye. The eye's gaze had to be directed through the exact center of the system in order for the spectacles to be effective. Any movement of the eye or head would produce intolerable distortion. Any movement of the body—even walking, rendered the system valueless. The usefulness of the spectacles, therefore, was limited to concentrated close work and fixed viewing at a distance—movies, television, sports spectacles, etc. Despite their tremendous boon

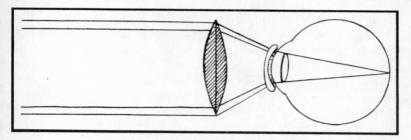

Fig. 86: The strong concave power is ground onto the contact lens and the strong convex objective power is in the form of a spectacle lens. The telescopic effect is the same.

to the partially-sighted, many did not take advantage of them because of these drawbacks.

The impracticality of these spectacles led to a new use for a contact lens—a lens which could overcome these deficiencies and be worn satisfactorily.

We remember that both the telescopic and microscopic systems required two lenses—an objective lens approximately 3/4ths of an inch in front of the eye, and an ocular lens nearer to the eye. If this ocular lens could be replaced by a contact lens only the objective lens would then have to be set before the eye. This could be mounted in a regular eyeglass frame. It would simply resemble a pair of ordinary glasses and still achieve the telescopic effect. Figure 86 shows the telescopic system with a contact lens as ocular.

This was tried years ago with scleral lenses and the early corneal lenses, but because of the difficulties encountered in fitting and wearing and the questionable effect on pathologically disturbed eyes, these efforts were never brought to a successful conclusion. Now, with a lens that was wearable and had no adverse effect on the eye, tests were resumed.

This time they were crowned with success. Frequent newspaper stories across the country described the transformation in the partially-sighted through the miracle of a contact lens-telescopic system. Restoration to ordinary pursuits—even obtaining a driver's license, has been the good fortune of many. One individual who had 20/100 with regular telescopic spectacles was improved to 20/30 with the contact lens-telescopic combination.

Aside from the obvious practicality of such a combination, visual betterment beyond the capability of a simple telescopic spectacle was not infrequent. The same reasons cited for improved vision in ordinary refractive defects with contact lenses seem to apply with greater force to a contact lens-telescopic combination.

In addition to the day-to-day use of today's vented lenses for the correction of routine and unusual refractive errors, for appearance sake, for sports and vocational reasons, there are additional advantages. They are plastic, they are practically unbreakable while worn and, as we have mentioned, require rare prescription changes.

We see that lenses have enlarged the capacity of refractive devices to remedy considerably visual abnormalities.

The professional person, the actor, the public speaker and the athlete have welcomed modern contact lenses as the most expedient refractive means for improved vision, without the need to sacrifice appearance or mobility.

Contact lens use has enjoyed a remarkable growth in recent years. More than six million persons in need of visual correction are gaining it through these tiny, almost-invisible aids to sight.

These then are the advantages and prospects of contact lenses in their modern vented form. We have explored them to their fullest.

Do the lenses have any disadvantages? And, if so, what are they?

The physiological disturbances reported by the Army Medical Study have been overcome. The effect of a contact lens on the eye is now thoroughly understood and if untoward can be corrected. Problems of application, removal and adaptation have been solved. Manufacturing processes too have achieved a much higher degree of perfection than at the time of the report. The precision of the modern vented contact lens meets the highest ophthalmic standards.

Other difficulties mentioned by the report—high cost, inadequate wearing-time, and uncommon skill required for fitting, have been removed by the following factors: The intensive codification and standardization of fitting of the vented lenses; the specialized instruments created for scientific fitting; the resultant reduction of fitting time and required visits to half the optimum needed by the Army's clinical staff; the heightened standard of living which today puts the modern vented lens within financial reach of the great majority.

The purely physical problems of durability or the greater ease with which plastic scratches as compared to glass are minor. The plastic used—plexiglass, it is true, scratches more easily, but care in handling will prevent this. Exposure tests proved the permanence of its optical qualities. After 200 days of full sunshine exposure there was less than a 1% decrease in transparency.

One factor not covered in the Army's report concerned the dryness property of the plexiglass, probably because wetting solutions were considered sufficient.

The Army's other point—the high motivation required by an individual to be fitted with contact lenses was very true then, but is perhaps not quite so true now. And this psychological factor leads us to perhaps the chief disadvantage—probably the only one, of modern-day contact lenses as a remedy for refractive error.

For this disadvantage is psychological in nature. Plainly, it is the fear of putting something into one's eye.

Actually this belief has no basis in fact. Lenses are never put "into" the eye—they are simply applied onto the eye and float on a fine layer of natural tear fluid.

No doubt this fear is based partly on experiences with the older type lenses. Compounding this fear is the extra care needed in applying contact lenses and the awareness of the presence of the lens during early stages of wear.

Physiologically it has been proven that there can never be a harmful effect on the eye with a modern, properly fitted and properly worn contact lens.

Psychologically, however, we have a problem which must be faced.

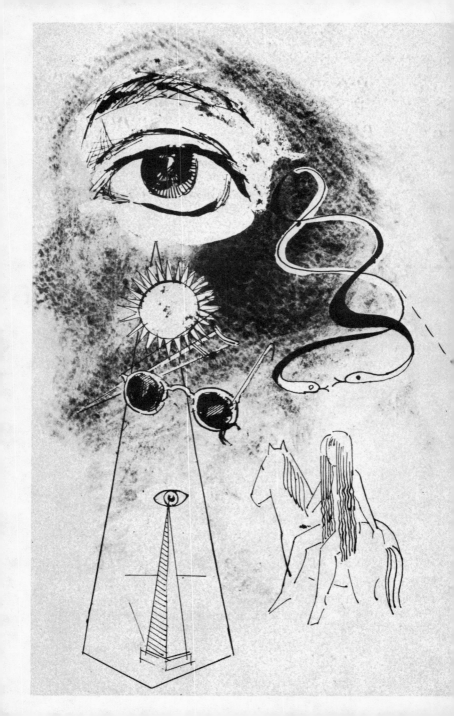

XIV

A New Look and a New Outlook

The fear that grips us when we think of any injury to our eyes is a very deep-rooted one.

It springs from the deep wells of childhood's teachings, admonitions and observations. It permeates all religion, literature and thinking. Next to life itself, next to survival, eyesight is our most treasured possession. Small wonder that fear immediately springs to mind when the eye is the subject.

Even everyday experiences—the trivial happenstance of a speck of dust catching under the lid—evoke a reaction completely disproportionate to the seriousness of the occurrence. Until the speck is removed, little else is important, and we have all known the tremendous feeling of relief which its removal occasions.

The reason for this is not hard to find. All our lives we have been impressed with the extreme sensitivity of the eye, although in truth it is one of the toughest and best protected organs of the body. Even in adulthood we find it difficult to overcome the unreasoning fear which the eye and its abnormalities provoke.

From a psychoanalytic point of view, it is not hard to symbolically equate the eye with what is considered the source of our basic drives—the sex organs. According to medical writers, psychoanalytic studies have revealed that the eye may symbolically represent either the male or the female genitals. The statement, "If I just look at her, she becomes pregnant," meaningful or not, seems to refer to the hypothetical beam of light emanating from the pupil of the eye as representing the penis.

The frequent allusions in legend, mythology, fairy tale, and even the Bible to the blindness visited upon those who gaze on forbidden sights (the Medusa, Sodom, Gomorrah) and the spells cast or removed through the agency of seeing, cannot be purely incidental. They point without question to the deep-rooted preoccupation with the eye as a sexual symbol, stemming from the very deepest primordial unconscious instincts—those self-same instincts which form the infantile fixations.

According to African bushman belief, the glance of a menstruating girl's eyes may affix a man in whatever position he may be at that precise moment and change him into a tree.

Legend tells us that Tiresias, the blind Greek seer, was blinded by Athena, the Greek goddess, because he saw her naked. In another legend, Tiresias saw two snakes coupling on Mount Cyllene. Instead of being blinded, he was deprived of masculinity and changed into a woman. Later on, seeing the same scene, he killed the male snake and became a man again.

Throughout legend and history the two seem intertwined—the eye and the sex organ—the fear of going blind and the fear of castration.

Modern psychiatry reveals cases where schizophrenic patients have been known to tear out both eyes and their testicles in self-castration as a penalty for fancied forbidden pleasures. Self-inflicted gouging out of the eyes as atonement for sexual excesses and aberrations is by no means uncommon.

It is related that in the early Christian era a young man became so captivated with the eyes of St. Lucy of Syracuse that he was unable to think of anything else. Lucy felt her vow of chastity was in danger, so she plucked out her offending eyes and sent them to him on a salver.

Even the famous tale of Oedipus is a case in point. Freud's theory of the Oedipus complex evolves directly from this legend—for Oedipus is fabled to have plucked out both his eyes because of incestuous relations with his mother.

The Sand-Man theme in the "Tales of Hoffman" is an apt illustration. In this tale the dreaded Sand-Man tears out children's eyes! Grains of sand are tossed into a child's eyes, which turn into red-hot grains of coal . . . sexual significance is not hard to find. That this is the true meaning of the Sand-Man fable, even in its harmless version today, requires little stretch of the imagination.

The saga of Lady Godiva is another instance. In this tale, Lady Godiva is forced to ride naked in broad daylight through the streets of a little town. To make her ordeal less painful, the inhabitants stay indoors and keep their windows shuttered. But one man peeps through the shutters at her nude beauty and is punished by becoming blind.

Freud further draws the eye as a dually functioning organ— both as a sensory organ and as a sexual component. His theory of hysterical blindness seeks to explain a loss of vision without an organic cause. He traces this blindness, as real as though physically caused, to a repression of vision due to a sexual conflict— simply put, something seen by the individual which according to the person's moral standard should never have been seen.

The middle of the forehead is known in psychiatry to frequently represent the genitals in fantasy, and it is legendary for one-eyed beings (the eye is in the middle of the forehead) to have been a source of dread and horror.

The eye's paramount place in eroticism is acknowledged, and aberrations deriving from this are recognized. Voyeurism—the visual gratification of sexual desire such as evinced by "peeping Toms," is a specific aberration. Exhibitionism—the deliberate exposure to view of the sex organs, is another. Both represent sublimations of the sex impulse to the visual sense.

Moreover, many present-day psychiatrists are prone to label the feelings many people have toward the blind as the mobilization or the embodiment of a castration fear.

Many ophthalmologists and psychiatrists find this so-called castration fear very real. Touching the eye in order to determine the presence of excessive hardness—as is done in glaucoma, is often a difficult maneuver for the ophthalmologist. Many patients will flinch and readily admit it is not pain but "the idea of touching their eyes" which is distasteful. A sexual significance is not hard to deduce.

In other ways, too, the effect and interplay of the eye and hidden emotion has been expressed and is present. For instance, the evil eye, the penetrating eye, the steely eye are referred to commonly as expressive of motion and psychological state. So are warm or soft eyes.

It is not surprising, therefore, that the eye has come to be regarded as somewhat apart from the other sense organs—something very special, something to be favored and certainly something to be fearful of and for.

With this background of understanding, we can see why, specifically, an individual might be afraid of contact lenses—why he might avoid a routine eye test—even why the average person resists any application of drops to his eye.

In a similar vein, we can see why someone would hesitate to encumber his eyes with ordinary eyeglasses. As a prime feature of expression—sexual or otherwise, it would appear that the eye should not be hidden or covered in any way. Yet if refractive error is uncorrected, strain and squinting usually manifest themselves and the normal appearance of the eye is altered. Attractiveness (to the opposite sex) may be diminished. The individual faces a dilemma. A psychological impasse is present.

Our story started with research indicating that eyeglasses were not a preferred way of correcting defective vision. These conclusions were based on practical rather than theoretical findings. Now we can be provided with a valid theoretical consideration—the psychological impasse which is quite possibly the prime motivating force in seeking other ways to correct vision.

Still other psychological influences surround the eyeglass wearer—such as the symbolism which eyeglasses may connote. Young children frequently want glasses to identify themselves with playmates or their brothers or sisters. To some, glasses may symbolize intellectual achievement or may be looked upon as a mark of distinction.

To others, glasses may provide a barrier or protection. Boys, for example, may want glasses to relieve them of fighting. Others hide behind dark glasses. Consciously or subconsciously, many will think of glasses in this vein.

On the psychosomatic level, eyeglasses appear to give tremendous relief in some cases of very minor refractive error. Without question the psychological benefit far outweighs the optical.

On the other side of the coin, however, there are the profound psychological disturbances which result from the wearing of glasses.

Every eye practitioner is well acquainted with many of the commonly assigned reasons why glasses are disliked and discarded. They are considered a cosmetic impediment; they signify age; and some types of prescriptions, such as strong convex or concave lenses, make glasses very unsightly.

Rarely mentioned, however, is the effect of glasses on personality. This is frequently a very pronounced one, since there is no doubt that many eyeglass wearers look upon their spectacles as a means of withdrawal and emotional support. Quite a common yet erroneous concept which intensifies this dependence on glasses is the belief that not wearing glasses when needed—or wearing the wrong glasses, can have a very serious effect on the eyes. Actually, there are no recorded cases where any damage has ever occurred.

It happens often, moreover, that this personality submersion —this subconscious dependency on glasses as a shield, becomes an integral part of an individual, and with the continuous wearing of glasses assumes a dominant role in his total outlook on life.

His participation in social activities, his leadership and fellowship roles, his business, professional or sports career—in fact every facet of his personal and family life is colored by wearing glasses. He does indeed feel, subconsciously or no, apart and different from the person who does not wear glasses.

Basically, of course, this feeling emanates from his innermost sense of having a bodily defect. In psychological terms, his body-image of himself is not a normal one. This innately abnormal body-image is fostered through his formative years by the attention and response which his visual defect draws from his immediate family, his friends, and his school environment. Later on in life it is supported by the reaction his wearing glasses elicits from the world around him, plus the handicaps and frustrations it may impose of itself.

The change in body-image which results from substituting contact lenses for glasses often brings about startling personality metamorphoses. The files of many eye practitioners abound with instances of these drastic changes occurring in individuals who finally discard their glasses.

A 23 year old girl had been wearing very thick glasses prescribed for congenital cataract since the age of 8. She was rather unattractive, poorly groomed and definitely had a withdrawn personality. Even wtih her glasses visual acuity was not better than 20/100, and she had been retarded in her school work and her employment because of poor vision. Needless to say, her social life was nil. Most regrettably, she was resigned to her unhappiness.

In her case contact lenses were advised. The change was astounding. Her vision, for one thing, improved to 20/25. Her eyes were open to view at last (and they were bright blue and attractive). Within two weeks—when she returned for her check-up, she was wearing a new outfit, her hair was done smartly, and cosmetics were used for the first time. She held her head up and walked erectly. She did not appear to be the same girl at all!

(Personal records.)

Not an uncommon story, by any means.
And witness the anecdote related in a popular magazine:

My friend, a striking blonde, had to show her license when she was stopped for a traffic violation. The officer read the description—Hair: Black, Weight: 125; Holder Must

Wear Corrective Lenses—then stared at my friend. "Whose license is this?" he demanded belligerently.

It took us the next half hour to convince him that since obtaining her license my friend had bleached her hair, taken off 20 pounds, and started wearing contact lenses.

(Readers Digest, June '59, p. 73, by MARY PERRY)

This particular story points up the "triggering" effect invisible vision correction has on upgrading appearance and personality.

These and other cases are instances where discarding glasses becomes the starting-point—the touchstone—for profound personality changes. Of course, if better vision is attained by invisible correction, the change in personality and outlook is even more pronounced than without better vision. But irrespective of this, the psychological handicap commonly imposed by glasses is effectively dispelled by these other means.

These theories have been confirmed in the course of motivational studies which particularly probed the pros and cons of contact lenses and the attitudes and impressions created in the average person's mind when he thinks of his eyes and contact lenses.

One survey uncovered the fact that of all eyeglass wearers interviewed not one would actually prefer to continue wearing glasses. Without exception, authoritative interviews disclosed that once the cover-up feelings of glasses as a protection or symbol are put aside, there was no eyeglass wearer who would not prefer to do without them. Nor did anyone agree with the view (if questioned sufficiently) that glasses might be becoming or would make one look better.

In many cases, mistaken ideas concerning the necessity of glasses and unsubstantiated opinions regarding other available means of eyesight correction were found to prevent an individual from discarding them.

That these latter mistaken ideas frequently color the modern eye practitioner's thinking as well has also served to deprive eyeglass wearers of the profound psychological benefits resulting from substituting some other means of eye correction. The average practitioner is well aware of the advantages of forms of visual correction other than glasses—but only from an optical point of view and only for specified visual defects. He overlooks or is entirely unfamiliar with the psychological factors.

Many instances are therefore encountered where eyeglass wearers are unknowingly discouraged—and unjustifiably so—from seeking the benefits of invisible lenses or forms of visual correction other than glasses.

Fortunately, increased public awareness of invisible sight corrective means such as contact lenses is taking place daily. Professional awareness of the psychological implications also is increasing. And increased newspaper, magazine, television and conversational reference to these modern-day means is making the subject more commonplace.

Most effective in the changing climate of awareness, of course, is the circle in which a new invisible lens wearer moves. Here there is no room for doubts and misconceptions—here is where the effect on the wearer's personality and outlook is easily discernible. Here is aroused the strongest motivation for others to move away from eyeglasses.

With particular reference to contact lenses, motivational studies have uncovered other explanations for the trend away from eyeglasses. Although in some respects some of these factors may be attributed to a "rationalizing" of the deep psychological urge to be free of glasses, they do reveal other influences.

For one, there is the purely utilitarian motive which cannot be minimized. Eyeglasses break and are a nuisance. Eyeglasses need frequent prescription changes. They have all the disadvantages cited with regard to weather and temperature. Because of these factors, the practical-minded eyeglass wearer would prefer a substitute.

Greater participation in sports—without glasses—is a definite factor. By whatever means obtainable, corrected sight without glasses is a very desirable plus to the visually defective participant in all types of sport.

For obvious reasons, glasses are simply impractical in certain professions and vocations. People who seek to enter these lines of work must find other means of visual correction. The theatrical performer, the model, the flyer or the seaman, and many others, must shun glasses. Many of these people are in the public eye, and hence their example is followed by many who seek to emulate them. Psychologically, then, glasses acquire an added aura of disfavor.

In summary, therefore, these are the findings confirmed by psychological and motivation studies:

... There are deep psychological reasons why an overt form of vision correction is undesirable.

... Not one wearer of eyeglasses would continue to wear them if he had an alternative means of vision correction.

... The innate fear of putting something into or near the eye can be dispelled by enlightenment.

... Ignorance of the newer forms of visual correction is as widespread as fear. Enlightenment here also is needed.

... Once fear and ignorance are removed, the alternative means of vision correction—particularly contact lenses, present other advantages apart from the psychological ones.

... Finally, the utilization of a means other than glasses to correct vision frequently leads to a complete blossoming of personality—indeed a new look and a new outlook.

IS THE EYE A SUPER-FRAGILE ORGAN?

CAN THE EYES BE DAMAGED BY OVERUSE?

IS "CLOSE-UP" WORK HARMFUL TO THE EYES?

IS BRIGHT LIGHT HARMFUL TO THE EYES?

DOES "DARKNESS" STRAIN THE EYES?

IS IT BAD TO READ IN BED?

IS TOUCHING THE EYE INJURIOUS?

CAN A CONTACT LENS GET "LOST" IN THE EYE?

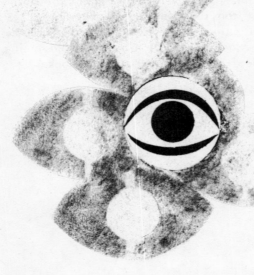

XV

Don't You Believe It

In our previous chapter we discussed the fear and ignorance which pervades the thinking of many on the subject of the eyes.

No survey of modern-day approaches to sight correction would be complete without an attempt to analyze and refute some of the misconceptions and irrational prejudices fear and ignorance have created . . .

One of the most widespread misconceptions concerns the physical status of the eye.

Is the belief that the eye is a hyper-fragile organ a valid one?

As we have noted, this concept is disproven by competent medical opinion. The eye is no more fragile, is in fact sturdier than most organs of the body. Aside from the excellent protection offered by the bony socket—as any prize fighter will attest—the eye itself is covered by tough fibrous layers encased in strong muscles.

The cornea possesses superlative powers of regeneration. The inside surface of the lids reacts effectively against irritation, infection or trauma. The high degree of sensitivity of nerve endings in these tissues is purely a protective device to quickly marshal the body's forces.

In general, the eye recuperates faster from irritation, trauma or infection than most organs of the body. The fear of permanent injury or blindness from everyday, normal activity is quite un-justified, and the danger of permanent vision impairment from serious or chronic affections has been materially reduced by modern ophthalmological therapy. The eye's apparently extreme sensitivity should not serve as an index of delicacy. Rather, it should be considered an otugrowth of natural conditioning.

What about the use of the eyes? What beliefs can be considered fact, and what ideas are pure fantasy?

In answering some of the more common questions about the eyes, it is our hope to set the record straight about the eyes and their workings.

Can the eyes be damaged or ruined by excessive use?

No amount of over-use or "strain" has ever been known to lead to anything more than transitory discomfort. Blindness or any organic eye disease has never occurred.

Is television viewing harmful to the eyes? Does close viewing indicate myopia?

Not so. Because most children, including those prone to myopia, adore magnification and enjoy the sense of involvement with the events on the screen. That's why children's books are in large print and most theaters for children are in the round. Scientific evidence points to the fact that prolonged television viewing on their part and then checking their eyes showed no correlation between the viewing and any muscular fatigue. A bright room makes the set more difficult to see, but doesn't ruin the eyes. A darkened room is not best either; and it's apparent that illumination determines comfort but plays no role in eye health.

Is close work of itself ruinous to the eyes?

Indeed not. Working under poor lighting conditions, wearing lenses with the wrong refractive correction—or no correction at all, may cause difficulty and discomfort—but never disease or organic damage.

Is bright light harmful to the eyes?

Only to the extent that it produces discomfort. The only truly damaging effect comes from staring directly into the sun or any source of ultra-violet light. And this rarely leads to blindness.

If an eye with impaired vision is used sparingly or not at all for any length of time, is vision conserved or retained?

Not at all. On the contrary, non-use of such an eye leads to further degeneration—even loss of vision. By using the impaired eye at maximum capacity, however, vision can possibly be retained and sometimes improved.

Does darkness strain the eye?

The eye is adapted by evolution to normal conditions of light—darkness and daylight. Darkness, therefore, is normal, and country dwellers such as farmers do not find darkness a strain on their eyes. By the same token, inhabitants of sunny countries do not find it necessary to wear dark glasses.

If one eye is used excessively (as by watchmakers), is it more likely to be strained or cause discomfort?

On the contrary. In such cases one of the prime causes of strain—the need for binocular vision, is eliminated. Actually, using just one eye produces less discomfort, if any, than when both are used.

Is touching the eye injurious?

Not of itself. Nor does the application of a therapeutic device such as a contact lens produce any adverse effect.

Will glasses, or other refractive correction, weaken your eyes so that you will never be able to do without them?

Obviously the answer is no. Most people see much better with their glasses or lenses than without them. They do not realize they had poor vision before they began to use corrective lenses. The contrast in vision when they take them off is so great that they believe their glasses have "weakened" their eyes.

This often happens with people who initially use glasses for reading (presbyopes). After some time has elapsed they find they cannot read comfortably without them. They forget they're simply growing older. Some thinking might regard eyeglasses, especially reading glasses, as "crutches," upon which the eye's lens and ciliary muscles grow to depend. Thus they lose their tonus as any unused muscle will.

The case comes to mind of a woman in her early seventies who came in stating, "It's time I had glasses." She said she'd avoided them by using bright lighting as soon as she noticed reading difficulty. Examination revealed her need for reading help—but she needed only about half what would have been normally expected. Evidently her not succumbing to an accommodative substitute, reading glasses, and her use of brighter lighting and larger print, had kept the eye muscles reasonably vigorous and had delayed the onset of presbyopia needing correction. This rationale itself is behind most eye practitioners' prescribing the least possible magnification for beginning presbyopia.

Will your eyes be harmed if you go without correction occasionally?

No. You won't see as well or as comfortably, but nothing else.

Is it bad to read in bed?

Not at all, if the lighting is adequate. Near-sighted children often read in bed, simply because they like to. This does not increase their myopia. If reading in bed had this effect, it would be welcomed as a form of treatment for far-sightedness!

Does wearing glasses once mean they can never be dispensed with?

Not at all. Many discard glasses after short periods of wear.

Do glasses have to be changed at fixed intervals?

Again, not at all. Some glasses never have to be changed, and only the wearer's own eye condition determines this. In any case, even though entirely unsuitable glasses may be worn, disease never develops. Glasses which are quite incorrect—even someone else's glasses—are worn without effect and, in many cases, without any discomfort whatsoever.

Must light be restricted in cases of certain diseases such as measles?

Not necessarily. Darkening of the room will not prevent soreness of the eyes in measles; it may, however, make the patient more comfortable if the eyes are already sore. During the treatment of certain eye diseases, bright light should not be allowed to fall directly upon the eyes.

Does a reduction in school work prevent the increase of near-sightedness?

Only to a limited degree, as is done in schools for the

partially-sighted or in sight-conservation classes. In general, myopia will increase to its natural peak whether school work is curtailed or not.

It seems to be a fairly well-accepted rule that a child's myopia will eventually approximate that of his parents if they are myopic —particularly if his age at onset is the same. If the myopia becomes evident earlier, it will probably exceed that of one or both parents. If the myopia appears later, it is likely to become less pronounced.

This does not take into account the effect of wearing the modern contact lens, which we have seen acts as a restraining influence on myopia. A generation or more of study will be needed on this to determine its long range effect.

The same heerditary influences appear to be present in other defects as well. Astigmatism is frequently traced from parent to child. Hyperopia likewise. And, of course, squint is very definitely linked to hereditary origin.

After a certain age, is it true that eyesight will get no better or worse?

Since we have seen that most defects of eyesight are structural in cause, it is obvious that only while eye structure is changing do these defects change. In the normal eye the front portion— the cornea, reaches its full growth at two years of age. The posterior portion of the eye continues to grow, however, until just before the teens. Usually, therefore, during this time the eye is somewhat far-sighted. Should the posterior portion continue to grow after this, near-sightedness is the result, as we have seen.

Once fully grown, however, the eye changes comparatively little and whatever defect is present remains fairly constant. Eyesight likewise is relatively unchanging. But in later years, at the time of presbyopia, the corneal surface does tend to flatten. This leads to astigmatism and also to increased hyperopia— which generally accompany presbyopia.

The fact that this corneal flattening is in most cases the only change in later years, aside from presbyopia, provides the reason why a contact lens—which replaces the cornea with a new, constant surface, so rarely needs changing.

Can color blindness be cured—by spectacles or any other means?

The nature of color blindness is still a mystery. And the various color theories shed no light on any method of preventing or curing it.

Does insufficient sleep lead to poor eyesight?

No more so than fatigue resulting from any other cause. The notion that eight hours of sleep is a physiological necessity has never been proven. Some people only require three or four hours, some feel tired if they do not get nine or ten. And the same individual at times may require only a few hours of sleep and at others can hardly get enough. The effect on the eye is no greater or less than on any other organ.

If one eye becomes inflamed or infected, is it true that the other eye will follow suit?

While it is true that certain cases occur where there appears to be a sympathetic reaction of the uninfected or uninflamed eye when its mate is affected, these are comparatively rare. With proper treatment and care there is little likelihood of this happening. Various theories to account for this rare occurrence are propounded.

Does sleeping in the moonlight produce blindness?

Of course not. The origin of this fable is obscure, but certainly moonlight has no deleterious effect on the eye.

Are cataracts an inevitable accompaniment of age? Or, to put it another way, would everyone get cataract if he lived long enough?

Presumably yes. One form of senile cataract is caused by the "sclerosing" or hardening process accompanying aging in lens tissues. The resulting opacity is usually less than from other forms, but definitely falls within the description of cataract. It requires advanced age and its development during a normal lifetime is generally regarded as an early or exaggerated senile manifestation.

Can cataract be cured by lemon juice?

Among the host of nostrums for various afflictions this is just another one. Medication of any form has very limited value insofar as controlling cataract. Surgery is still the only sure remedy.

Should an operation for cataract be delayed until the cataract is ripe, i.e., fully mature?

As a general rule, taking into consideration the actual visual impairment of the affected eye and the visual status of the other eye, most ophthalmologists will follow this rule of thumb.

Are drops necessary to test vision?

Only in certain cases where there might be excessive activity of the accommodative muscles which would obscure the defect—high hyperopia in children, for instance—would drops be required. They are also used where the pupil must be dilated for a better view of the back of the eye. So far as measuring the structural defect of the eye, drops will give no greater accuracy.

Theoretically, a wider pupil would produce a shorter depth of focus and therefore a narrower range of clear vision—just as a dilated aperture in a camera would do. Glasses prescribed, therefore, from a patient's subjective visual appreciation when a pupil is dilated would appear to be more accurate than those spectacles prescribed when the pupil is constricted. Practically speaking, however, since objective means are also used, the difference is negligible. And there are certain conditions—such as glaucoma —where drops would definitely not be desirable.

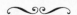

Insofar as the more modern forms of visual correction are concerned, for the most part they have not been with us long enough for misconceptions and prejudices to have been awakened.

In the case of contact lenses, however, many misunderstandings have arisen—some based on the older, unsuccessful scleral types which have contributed to the psychological impediments we have discussed, and others revolving about the newer, corneal type. These are some of the typical questions.

Can a corneal contact lens fall behind the eye?

This is impossible. The under-surface of the eyelids forms a continuous membrane which turns and becomes the outer surface layer of the eyeball itself—the conjunctiva. At no point is there any opening behind the eye—the lids and the eye itself form a closed chamber through which nothing can penetrate.

Don't corneal contact lenses slip out of place—off the center of the eye?

Since the curvature of the lens corresponds with the corneal curve of the eye, and this is a great deal more curved than the scleral part, it is very unlikely that this will happen except, perhaps, during application. When it does happen, it will move by itself until it becomes recentered on the cornea.

Does crying interfere with proper functioning of contact lenses?

No. The tear glands are situated upward and outward from the eye and the flow of tears is downward towards the nose. They will flow uninterruptedly over and under the lens, without displacing it in any way.

Can one swim with contact lenses?

This depends on the individual and the conditions. The normal tightness of the lids, the roughness of the water, and the amount of eye movement will determine whether it is advisable to wear lenses while swimming.

If someone is struck in the eye while wearing a contact lens, would the lens break or damage the eye?

Quite the contrary. A case does not come to mind of a contact lens broken while being worn—and many cases where it has shielded and protected the eye from serious injury. Unless dropped and crushed, the plastic used in modern-day contact lenses is virtually unbreakable.

If you happen to fall asleep with lenses on, would anything serious happen?

No. Many people will nap with their lenses on. Although people have been known to wear them while sleeping and some even for weeks and months without removal, it is generally recommended that they be removed while sleeping. This is to refresh and rest the eye.

Can you smile when you are wearing contact lenses?

Oddly enough, this is a question many have asked. Some people have the impression that the eyes (and the face) must be held rigid or else the lenses would float out of place. Of course, this is not so. The heartiest laughter can be indulged in. Once properly in place there is little chance the lenses will change position.

Can contact lenses change the color of your eyes?

Yes, although it is more difficult to make brown eyes blue than blue eyes brown. Dark green contact lenses are being widely used to screen out the glare of the sun.

Do contact lenses cause cancer or cataract?

No. There have never been any cases of cancer or cataract reportedly caused by contact lenses.

And probably the most comprehensive question of all:

Can everyone wear contact lenses?

No. Most people can—because their eyes are healthy and they are adequately motivated. There is the occasioanl exception—an individual whose eyes may not be healthy or who may be psychologically unprepared or simply too sensitive.

There very likely are other questions and doubts—not only about contact lenses and the newer forms of vision correction, but about eyes and eye health in general. These, as mentioned before, are the outgrowth of centuries of conditioning—they have their origin in legend, mythology and old wives' tales, and in many cases can barely be expressed.

A fresh, new look at the subject should serve to clear away some of the cobwebs of superstition and ignorance surrounding the eyes. Enlightenment on the newer methods of eye correction—on drug and vitamin therapy, on surgery, on visual exercises and contact lenses should prevent similar bugaboos from developing with respect to these methods.

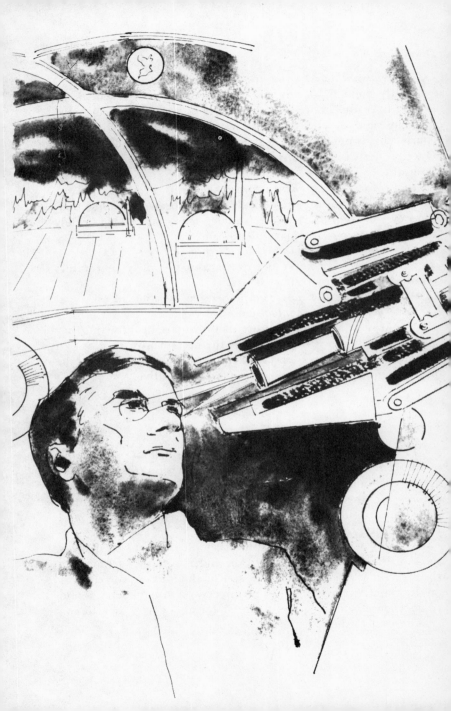

XVI
What Does the Future Hold

The place of a prophet is indeed a precarious one.

Yet when one sees the remarkable advances made so rapidly in practically all branches of science—bringing to actuality theories just a few years old, it is hard to refrain from offering predictions.

When one has witnessed the startling forward steps mere decades have brought, the future possibilities for eye treatment and correction appear particularly bright.

What will happen in the processes of the eye's natural evolution over coming thousands of years, as well as the changes which may be wrought by radioactive mutation, elude prediction.

Theory and conjecture hold that in future civilizations, as we become more and more dependent on our eyes, our heads will tend to become larger in proportion to our bodies. Our other senses will dull and atrophy much as the sense of smell already has. Our eyes will eventually become the dominant features in our heads. Our brains will then become more and more receptors and storehouses for optical images and memories.

Biological exploits which include the artificial production of monsters by X-ray and chemical means may well advance the art of grafting and transplantation . . . so much so that a complete eye may replace a diseased or defective one. The origin of this is seen in present-day experiments on primitive eyes. A recent one entailed grafting the eye of a salamander on to the body of a newt. The transplanted eye begins to function again,

perceiving, seeing, reacting to light . . . and though the salamander's eye has less sharpness of vision than the newt's, when
it is transplanted it still sees better than it did in its original
host!

In other respects, too, the distant future holds a promise of
possibilities which are hardly fantastic. Color vision in the
human eye is recognized to be unique and far-advanced. Yet ages
ago the range of color in the spectrum visible to the human eye
very likely was much narrower than it is today. In the future
the sensitivity of the eye may have heightened to include a still
broader range—the infrared and below, the ultra-violet and
above, removing these radiations from the non-visible bands
they now occupy.

Unquestionably, the eye will retain its functions as an
optical system for many millenia to come. Yet who knows how
much greater its resolving power may be, how much more
accurate its space perception, its focusing, its sensitivity may
become.

The age of space travel which is upon us will bring attendant
problems of communication and navigation. Who knows to what
extent trained, skilled eyesight—far more than the other senses—
may prove a selective factor of survival. And what special training devices to achieve this advanced eyesight will have been
created . . . devices which may well banish refractive error.

Fantastic? Not really. Certainly no more improbable than
was radioactivity a mere century ago.

The immediate future, though, permits more valid conjecture. Looking about us today we can readily envisage the paths
of research and how future studies will affect sight and sight
correction.

In one direction—that of medical knowledge, the path leads
to increasingly potent anti-infective agents, both chemical and
antibiotic. What this will mean in the expanded utilization of
surgery—by removing its chief enemy, one rejoices to hypothesize.

New applications in the surgical treatment of retinal detachment, in glaucoma and cataract are inevitable. Combating

myopia by reducing the depth of the eyeball by surgery may well follow. The more prosaic replacement of defective eye structures —the cornea, the crystalline lens—by methods and with materials more effective than today's corneal transplants and lens inserts— is virtually a certainty.

Modern ophthalmological research is uncovering the interplay of general bodily conditions, glandular activities, and emotional and mental attitudes as contributors to visual anomalies. The individual's reaction to stress and strain is being assigned its due responsibility. As these factors are understood, more efficient therapy to control them will be devised. Consequently, visual defects and affections they engender will decline.

Research on specific drugs—such as adrenaline and atropine— which truly inhibit myopia, is currently in progress. Dietary supplements which greatly improve eye health and lessen the eye's proclivity to defects are already in the picture. The medical treatment of progressive eye conditions such as cataract is continually being bettered. Glaucoma is gradually becoming less of a mystery. In addition to surgery, drug therapy for relieving and curing this disease is advancing.

In another direction—the physico-chemical one, research is taking ever bolder steps.

From time to time experiments are conducted designed to short-circuit the eye—to circumvent it completely—by stimulating optic nerve impulses by electronic rather than optical means. In a way this bears a resemblance to television—a mere dream fifty years ago, which utilizes electronic impulses to produce light images.

The case is cited of a New Jersey woman, blind for 18 years, who experienced vision—actual optical imagery. This was accomplished by excitation of the inactive optic nerve with an electronic impulse. Theoretically this hardly seems difficult. Yet the problem of creating recognizable images in such a manner presents a great challenge. No more so, however, than did television short years ago.

It is entirely within the range of possibility, then, that an electronic camera may in certain cases substitute for the eye's entire refractive apparatus!

The use of a photo-electric cell connected to the brain by tiny wires has been attempted in other experiments with the blind. Flashes of light are recorded and transmitted by the photo-electric cell. The blind person receives a definite perception of the direction and intensity of these flashes. He can be said to see them!

One conclusion drawn from these experiments is that long unused brain cells do not lose their receptive power as do unused muscles, and that other brain cells may usurp the function of damaged ones . . . conclusions extremely important to other research in this direction.

Where brain damage is not involved, this electronic approach, of course, offers infinite promise to the totally blind. When blindness is due to interference with light transmission through the eye (opacity) —corneal destruction, inoperable cataract or even retinal detachment, such an electronic eye will enable an individual to distinguish light from dark and ultimately, it is to be hoped, form and motion.

Further, it is not difficult to conceive of the use of electronic lenses to supplement the eye's optical system in the near-blind. Such lenses would magnify or reduce image size electronically. Already an increase or decrease of light intensity has been accomplished by electronic means. The recording of television video portions on tape rather than on film seems a long forward step in this direction.

In more commonplace ways the future holds promise of great improvement in diagnosis—to determine the causation of eye defects and abnormalities and the actual physiological changes involved. Greater understanding of the photo-chemical reactions of light and the effect of nonvisible radiations is bound to come. The true chemical and tissue changes in keratoconus, corneal dystrophy and cataract are bound to be revealed.

Better instrumentation—such as the corneascope—for the measurement of eye refraction and the surfaces composing the eye's optical system, must of necessity lead to more accurate correction of defects. Aniseikonia should be corrected as easily as astigmatism.

Newer defects—or old defects more correctly identified—may become increasingly prevalent. Polymorphopsia, images appearing in different shapes; metamorphopsia, images apparently changing shape; polyopia, the seeing of several images of the same object—all ascribed to differences of refraction within the same refractive medium, may be added to our classic four refractive errors. Who knows what internal eye changes may take place with the many potent drugs and hormone extracts which will be administered?

Some modern theories hold that near-sightedness itself is civilization's response to increased close work. They maintain that the eye is slowly changing in basic structure as part of an evolutionary process, so that it can adapt more easily to the near tasks required now and in the future.

Certainly it is true that the myopic eye places a far lesser demand on its accommodative powers. The nearsighted person is generally more comfortable at reading without any artificial aid than his far-sighted or even his normal-sighted brother. Not only that but, because so little accommodation is required, near-sightedness sometimes delays the onset of manifest presbyopia indefinitely.

Whether this is really nature's adjustment, and whether myopia will become more and more accepted as the normal rather than the abnormal, coming centuries will tell. It may well be that the norm of visual acuity at some future date will be 20/100 rather than 20/20, and the eye will have reached another level in its evolutionary ascent!

Be that as it may, inevitably the future will lead to the greater application of visual training and exercise. Problems of binocular coordination, squint and muscular insufficiency, will be diagnosed earlier and corrected at inception. Incorrect visual habits will be halted and changed sooner. Conceivably the increasing use of visually stimulating exercises will lead to the quicker counteracting of amblyopia and greater refinement of visual acuity. Evolution may well compound this refinement.

Along this avenue, standards of vision may become—instead of 20/400 to 20/20—20/100 to 20/5. The true nature of the crystalline lens' accommodation will be revealed . . . the physiological aging which causes its gradual diminution may be controlled and delayed by therapy presently unknown . . . the onset of presbyopia may be deferred as our life span is increased.

The greater understanding of color, increasing daily, will most likely be put to use in making visual tasks easier and in making refractive errors less bothersome, much as present tentative experiments indicate that red light is refracted less than green. It would be logical to find that the far-sighted person, therefore, sees better under green light, and the near-sighted one under red.

Finally, one must mention the great promise the future holds for the contact lens. It is hardly unlikely that within the very near future this almost invisible lens will be worn constantly—never requiring removal or replacement.

When that day comes, the contact lens will need merely be applied once and thereafter removed only for very special reasons. Its further use in routine cases of refractive defect, as well as in subnormal vision needs, is well-nigh inevitable.

Very little of what has been said here is in the realm of fantasy or even imagination—some are projects already in the experimental and laboratory stages.

Surely the steps to the realization of these goals are no greater than those already trod to bring us to the great advancements in visual correction we have today . . . a far cry from the poultices and crystals of ancient times, the collyria, couching operations and spherical spectacles of medieval days, and even the precision ophthalmic eyeglasses of yesteryear.

XVII

The Future Unfolds

In the years that have passed since our last chapter was written, many of the predictions and hopes have begun to be realized. For one thing, the electronic imagery envisioned to replace sight for the blind or enhance it for the near-blind has seen some concrete developments.

Back in 1961, it was forecast by a noted Israeli physicist and electronics engineer that electronic devices would soon bring "light to the blind and hearing to the deaf." He predicted that blind persons would carry photoelectric cells and the deaf would be equipped with microphones that would "by-pass dead eyes and ears and transmit sight and hearing directly to the brain by an electrochemical process."

The scientist explained that vision was normally caused by the effect of rays of light upon cells in the retina. The rays perturb the ions, which send small electric impulses to the brain where they register sight. He said he had ascertained mathematically what happened in terms of theoretical physics when light entered the retina and sound the inner ear. "The photoelectric cells that blind persons will carry will be the same as those that convert natural pictures into electric impulses in television cameras.

"A blind person will be able to see something coming against him, but he will not know whether it's a car or a human being. He will not be able to distinguish shapes. That will require further development over a long period."

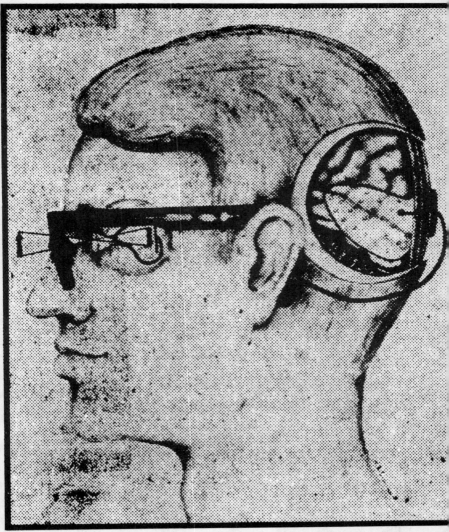

Fig. 87: As in artist's conception, researchers hope that ultimately many blind will be able to see by means of subminiature TV camera in glass or plastic eye and computer in spectacle frame. Signals would go to tiny transmitter at back of head and be picked up by an implanted receiver connected to electrodes in the visual cortex of the brain.

This research was the genesis of continuing exploration. But it was not until more than a dozen years later that further development was recorded.

In 1974 at a prominent American university, a team of researchers reported the successful elicitation of artificial sight in two blind patients, one of whom had seen nothing for twenty-eight years.

The two patients, one twenty-nine years old and one forty-three, were enabled to see dots of light by the stimulation of an array of electrodes implanted in the visual cortex of their brains. The electrodes were connected by cable to television cameras, with the system bypassing the retina, the optic nerve, and the ocular mechanisms by which the sighting process evokes images in the brain (Fig. 87).

Both men were involved in the project for at least four years. Grids of sixty-four electrodes were implanted at the back of their heads and it was noted that if the electrodes were all stimulated at the same time they would look like a sky full of stars. Only

---

THE NEW YORK TIMES, Sunday, April 2, 1961.

Electronic 'Eyes' for the Blind Are Sought by Israeli Scientist

Photoelectric Cells Would Flash Light to Brain— Aid for Deaf Is Seen

Special to The New York Times.

HAIFA, Israel, April 1—A noted Israeli physicist and electronics engineer has forecast that electronic devices will soon bring light to the blind and hearing to the deaf.

Prof. Franz Ollendorf of the Israel Institute of Technology here said that blind persons would carry photoelectric cells and the deaf would be equipped with microphones that would by-pass dead eyes and ears and transmit sight and hearing directly to the brain by an electrochemical process.

He warned, however, that he had no hope of affording full vision to the blind. He will be

---

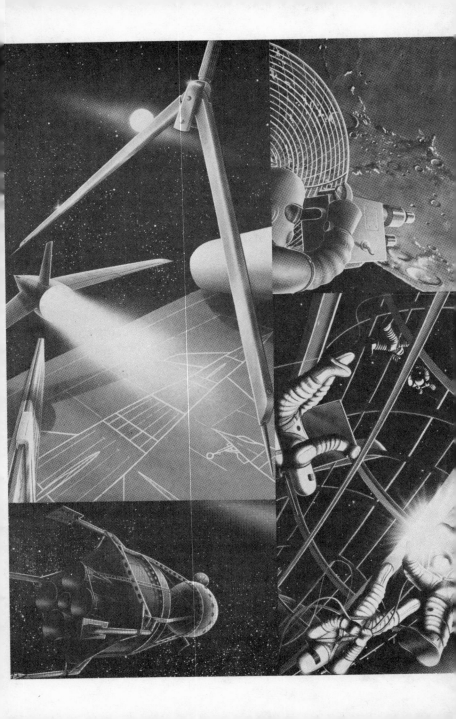

some of the electrodes were stimulated simultaneously, however, creating a pattern such as a square or a reversed letter "L."

The younger patient, who was blinded in Vietnam several years prior, could detect the pattern; the older could see the dots, called phosphenes, but, the report said, could not make out the patterns. During the experiment the electrodes were stimulated for about one second at a time. The stimulation period was short because one of the unknown factors is how much such stimulation will affect the brain and how the brain tissue will affect the electrodes, which are made of platinum and Teflon.

In transmitting the message to the electrodes, the researchers first selected a pattern which is projected on a TV screen as dots of light. The computer then stimulates the electrodes in a manner corresponding to the dots of light on the screen. The patient could detect the pattern and then mapped it successfully.

When the instrumentation is all completed, the researchers advise, it will consist of a miniature TV camera placed in an artificial eye in the eye socket. The camera will be attached to a mini-computer situated in the frame of eyeglasses. The computer will then process the light impulses and pass them along to a transmitter placed just under the scalp, camouflaged by hair. Another instrument, a receiver, will be placed under the skull and will be connected to the electrodes in the visual cortex.

It is hoped that by a complicated decoding process in the computer, the brightness of the dots can be adjusted so that, taken together, they can form a picture much like newspaper pictures which are made up of varying sizes of dots.

A simpler system, with a TV camera hooked directly into a computer, rather than into an artificial eye in turn hooked to the computer, is announced in the daily press (*N.Y. Post,* 8/5/74, p. 22). Computer stimulation of sixty-four pinpoint electrodes implanted in the portion of the brain controlling vision produced specks of light allowing the blind wearer to "read" vertical and horizontal Braille characters, five times faster than can be done by touch.

In the words of the wearer, "The spots of light I saw were about the size of a softball. Most of them were red. One looked

NEW YORK POST, Thursday, January 22, 1976.

Blind Man Is Plugged Into Computer & 'Sees'

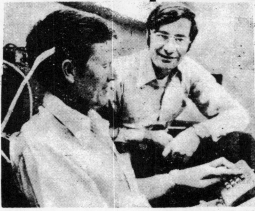

Associated Press Wirephoto

A blind man sees, thanks to a computer hooked up to his brain. Dr. Michael G. Mladejovsky is conducting the research.

By DAVID BRISCOE

SALT LAKE CITY (AP) — A 33-year-old man blind for a decade can read braille five times as fast now that he can "see" it with the help of a computer he plugs into his brain, scientists say.

Scientists also said yesterday that the man has been able to recognize vertical and horizontal lines through a small television camera hooked into the computer.

"I never expected anything like it. I was just overwhelmed. It's hard to explain," said the patient, describing his experience last August, the first time he had seen light in 10 years.

The experiments are the latest developments in a $1-million artificial vision project. A research team from the universities of Utah and Western Ontario, Canada, developed the program.

Details were released Wednesday by the project's director, Dr. William H. Dobelle, head of the University of Utah Neuroprostheses Program. The announcement followed publication of the experiments in the British scientific journal "Nature".

Dobelle said the research eventually could lead to development of a miniature computer in the frame of a pair of glasses that would be used to convert images seen by an eye socket camera into artificial sight. Dobelle declined to estimate when such devices would be available, but he said they would probably cost between $3,000 and $5,000.

The lights Craig now sees are produced by computer stimulation of 64 pinpoint electrodes implanted on the portion of his brain which controls vision. The platinum electrodes are connected by a tube to a quarter-size socket camouflaged under his hair. A computer programmed to produce braille images is then plugged into the socket.

The braille alphabet normally consists of six raised dots in different configurations. For Craig, the dots are specks of light, which allow him to read about 30 characters a minute, five times faster than he can by touch, Dobelle said.

Craig compared what he sees with time and temperature signs or the numbers on a football scoreboard. He said at times the lights also look "like distant stars".

"The phonemes (spots of light) I saw in the operating room were about the size of a softball. Most of them were red. One looked just like the moon. A few were yellow and one was real gold. They had the most pretty colors I believe I've ever seen, just as clear as could be . . . just beautiful," he said.

Reprinted by permission of the Associated Press.

just like the moon. A few were yellow and one was real gold. They had the most pretty colors I believe I've ever seen, just as clear as could be . . . just beautiful." But most beautiful of all was the fact that perception of light was evoked and, as mentioned, previews the commercial development of a miniature computer in the frame of a pair of eyeglasses which would be used to convert images seen by an eye socket camera into artificial "sight." And the *Post* (1/22/76, p. 5) followed up the story.

Thus a device is envisioned which would enable the wearer to see outlines of letters well enough to read and outlines of objects well enough to walk with safety—at least to the point of allowing a blind person to walk out of a room without bumping into things and go to the men's room without accidentally entering the ladies' room. What has been demonstrated so far is that even though eyesight is lost, the brain's potential for vision remains intact.

The number of people who could be helped by such an instrument, if perfected, is unclear. There are about 110,000 people in Canada and the U.S. who are totally without useful sight and three times that number who are considered "legally blind" (vision below 20/400), according to the above report. Estimates are offered that the miniature device, if it can be developed, would not sell for less than $5,000. But it is believed such a boon would quickly be underwritten by Federal funds.

On a less dramatic level, although perhaps of more immediate benefit to more individuals, have been the advances in electronic and computer technology relative to corneal measurement. These led to progress in the tracing of keratoconus (p. 127) and also to measurement of corneal dimensions most helpful to the contact lens fitter.

Advancing from the Corneascope (p. 161) probably the pioneer instrument of its kind, a device called the Photo-Electronic Keratoscope was introduced in the late '60s and improved in the early '70s. Essentially it was a camera, like the Corneascope, about

2 feet long and 14 inches in diameter. It used a xenon flash to make a sort of topographical picture of the patient's cornea (Fig. 88).

The photograph is developed automatically in 10 seconds and is then sent for computer processing after 50x enlargement. The conventional corneal-measuring instrument, the keratometer (p. 159) can span slightly over 3 mm. (about 1/8th of an inch) of the average 11 to 12 mm. cornea whereas the new P.E.K. succeeded in recording a corneal diameter of 10 mm. Further, although the keratometer measures variations as little as ¼ of a Diopter (unit of lens strength) P.E.K. was reported to measure down to 1/100th D.

Minute variations in corneal curvature, important to fitting lenses to highly distorted eyes, could then be transmitted to a computer and a contact lens produced with the eye's curvature and prescription automatically (Fig. 89). In post-cataract fitting, particularly where irregularity has been created by the surgery,

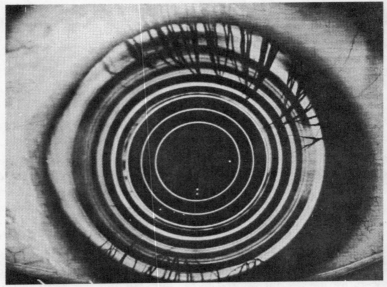

Fig. 88: Photokeratogram of the normal cornea.

photographic accuracy and computer reproduction is most helpful.

In essence the procedure is to place the patient in front of the P.E.K. He is told to look into the device and focus on a target surrounded by concentric circles of light. These rings are reflected onto his cornea and the variations of the corneal surface distort the perfect circles. In the words of one medical writer (J. Osterhoudt of the Newark *Star-Ledger*, 2/6/72, p. 37) , "The new technique is similar to that used in topography, where an aerial photo of a land surface can be used to accurately compute the variations in height and contours of the land." It is this distorted reflection which is photographed. The system uses a Polaroid camera, as the Corneascope initiated, which develops the film in ten seconds. In the laboratory, these photographs are blown up and measurements are fed into a computer which, by comparing them to the known measurements of the concentric circles, gives the corneal dimensions.

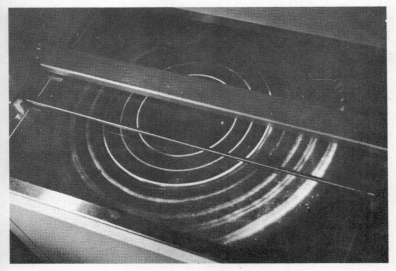

Fig. 89: Reading device for digitizing the photokeratogram. (Courtesy, G. L. Feldman, Ph.D.)

The patient's prescription is also fed into the computer and the final printout gives the exact specifications to which the lenses are to be ground. This advancement, it is claimed, makes it possible for an increased percentage of eyeglass wearers to be fitted for contact lenses. So far as P.E.K.'s utilization to measure any loss of reflectivity as indicated with the Corneascope (p. 162), as yet no data has been assembled or released on this subject, but it certainly remains within theoretical calculation and practical accomplishment.

Concurrently, too, there has been the utilization of modern computer technology in the programming and processing of corneal data obtained quite apart from electronic photography— all to the refinement of contact lens fitting.

XVIII

Enter the Computer

The limitation of the ophthalmometer (keratometer) alluded to on p. 159 nowhere became more apparent than in the years which saw the increased use of the vented lens. Between the vents, the lens' peripheral inside surface ideally should conform to the cornea's curvature there. But here was where the cornea's surface flattened out (Fig. 75B).

For many years, therefore, an approximated curvature was used in grinding this part of the lens. It was arbitrarily flatter than the central curve, actually a first, second, or third bevel depending on the lens size. And this estimated curvature was spherical, because no way had yet been found to grind any other on the inside of the lens even if the cornea could have been measured at its outer rim.

Finally, in the early '70s, a method was devised using an adaptor on the keratometer permitting the fitter to take peripheral corneal readings. Still only an approximated, spherical reading of a surface which was not spherical. This second reading was called "K_2" as distinguished from the first, central reading "K_1" (Fig. 90), and the procedure was in two stages.

The second stage involved feeding both K_1 and K_2 readings into a sophisticated, high-speed computer, much as figures from the P.E.K. photo were fed. This computer was programmed for a gradual transition from K_1 to K_2 and computed the grinding curvature needed in the finished lens. At the same time it made an allowance for a microscopically thin layer of tears between the

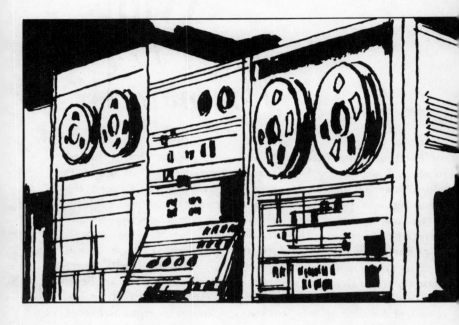

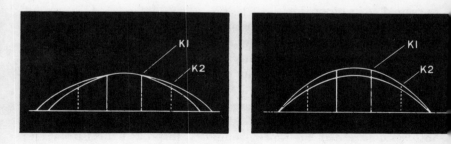

Fig. 90: Since present K_1 readings only measure 6 to 8% of the surface area of the cornea, it is obvious that the K_2 reading now gives the fitter an accuracy factor heretofore impossible to achieve. (Courtesy Compucon Co.)

lens and the cornea. This is necessary for proper tear flow and oxygen intake.

The final print-out included size of lens, its prescription, thickness, etc., with error claimed to be no more than ± four millionths of a millimeter—truly remarkable precision.

It was demonstrated that the gradual inside flattening of the lens, from its central to its peripheral curve, permitted better reading and use at near for the older wearer. Its effect was a bifocal one as the wearer looked down and the lens shifted slightly upwards (pp 151-52).

The improvement in near vision with such a lens was caused by the fact that the flatter a lens's inside curve is, the stronger the magnification becomes. In the words of one manufacturer, "this . . . is a magnificent precision grind that gives the beautiful vision contained in the blend between the two distances, so that . . . vision goes from the center for distance, the in-between vision . . . used for reading across a desk, shopping, card-playing, to the near for close reading, make-up, typing, etc."

A lens of this multi-focal nature raised obvious speculation as to its particular value in "myopia reduction"—the tantalizing prospect (pp. 172-75) of controlling and even diminishing near-sightedness. The use of weaker concave lenses than the myopia required, the "crowding of the plus," as professional parlance had it, and the bifocals prescribed for the nearsighted teenager to reduce any accommodative spur—all these were accepted parts of ophthalmological and optometric practice. Indeed, even the peripheral bevels of a concave contact lens were now seen to have a likely "plus" effect at close work for the teen-age myope and might be a considerable factor in arresting or reducing myopia. This concept now received new impetus from the computerized grinding process—but let us examine the whole rationale more fully.

"Developmental," as distinguished from patently inherited, myopia has been found to be restrainable. Known also as "acquired," "progressive," or "school" myopia, this is defined as a nonhereditary nearsightedness acquired as a result of continued near-point environment. Progression is usually between the ages of 5 and 25. In these ages, myopia may increase from approximately 4 percent at ages 4 through 11 to 50% of all student tested at high school and college age.

In contrast, a study performed on some Alaskan Eskimos revealed a non-myopic development due to outdoor exposure. Parents and grandparents had no schooling at all and spent their time hunting, fishing and doing nondemanding near work. Children had compulsory schooling. When these children's vision was compared to that of the nonschooled adults, the results were conclusive for the theory of developmental myopia. 51% of the children showed significant myopia—none of the adults did. Monkey studies, too, have had their environments limited to 24″ or less. Moderate myopia was created. And there is also the observation that continual driving with a spotted, unclear windshield will induce some nearsightedness. The value, therefore, of distance viewing to prevent myopia or counteract myopic tendencies cannot be gainsaid; in fact, the hero of *Two Years Before The Mast,* in the story written in the mid-1800s, undertook his long voyage for this very reason.

How can we prevent or correct this form of myopia? 1) **Reg**ular eye examinations including both external and internal eye muscles. These correlate the effort to focus on near objects with the eyes' turning in to maintain single vision. 2) Proper environmental conditions—adequate lighting and avoidance of undue reflection from reading matter. 3) Help by the use of slightly magnifying lenses if they seem beneficial. These inhibit the accommodative stress, the near focusing, and prevent fatigue which can lead to myopic progression.

Since part of this progressive myopia is due to excessive eyestrain at near work, the eyes' turning in for single vision may cause, it is alleged, pulling on the cornea and hence an increase in its curvature. This induced increase could be counteracted by properly applying pressure from a contact lens, it was theorized, and the myopia could be arrested quite apart from the lens' proven clarity, more normal image size, greater field of vision, and then unrealized peripheral relief-of-focusing effect, due to the gradual center-to-edge lens flattening already noted.

The science of "Orthokeratology" was thence born. Literally it meant "cornea-straightening." Its alleged accomplishments have been to reduce or arrest myopia by wearing successively flatter and flatter contact lenses. Firm physical pressure would cause the central corneal curve to flatten itself. From full-time to intermittent day-time wear, then merely to part-time wear terminating with the use of a retainer lens occasionally—this is the standard procedure. There is claimed to be no permanency in the ostensible reduction of myopia, merely a retention of results if proper procedures are followed. Generally a year or more would be consumed in the program and weekly or biweekly visits scheduled.

The procedure, however, has gained sparse medical acceptance, so further experimentation and controlled research is sorely needed. Inconsistently, too, even contact lenses fit more curved than the cornea have produced this myopia-reduction effect on occasion; and, similarly, cases of far-sightedness, where the cornea may be too little curved, have reportedly enjoyed a hyperopia reduction with contacts. The subject, therefore, is far from an established therapy. The belief is more and more confirmed that contact lenses, by their inherent advantages, may very well of themselves have this ameliorative effect on all visual anomalies. And perhaps the best advice for one contemplating this orthokeratological program is that medical check-ups of the corneal epithelium be had at frequent intervals.

Naturally, the rigidity of the contact lens being the purported agent of the corneal flattening, it was inevitable that the question be raised as to the place of the nonrigid or flexible lens in the program, if it had a future and the lens's place for all other contact lens purposes as well.

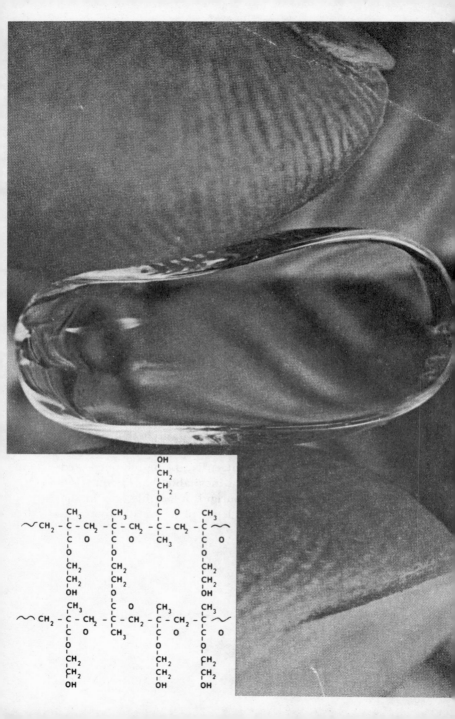

XIX

The Soft Lens and Its Aftermath

Sir John Herschel's idea to use transparent gelatin in contact with the eye to correct irregular astigmatism (p. 123) had kept burrowing at the minds of scientists since it was expressed. A contact lens with its inner surface filling in the cornea's deformities, and its outer surface correcting the eye's defect, was a far-out concept which never materialized . . . until . . .

In the early 1960s, experiments were conducted with a plastic newer than the poly-methyl-methacrylate (PMMA) then and currently used for contact lenses. One of the important reasons was the dryness of the outer surface of the PMMA which surfaced when the problem of edge sensation was resolved. (p. 149) The new plastic was called "Hydron" and was hydrophilic (water-loving). Hydro-ethyl-methacrylate (HEMA) was its chemical designation. It was developed in Czechoslovakia by two chemists, Dr. C. Wichterle and Dr. D. Lim.

The new material was hard and transparent. It could be cut, ground, or molded into a variety of shapes and had virtually the same refracting power as PMMA. It seemed chemically inert and fully compatible with human tissue. And it could be ground to inside and outside curvatures just as PMMA. Its chief distinction was its ability to absorb water and swell to approximately twice its volume while retaining its basic curvatures. This seemed a natural for contact lenses, being pliable and form-fitting when wet, and above all being hydrophilic so dryness would not be a problem.

The difficulty was that the lenses took up water like a sponge and, instead of permitting oxygen exchange, retained the water "like a stagnant swamp," in the words of one ophthalmologist. Vision through it was quite hazy. Also, the design was such that the cornea beneath was starved for oxygen and consequently swelled.

Despite these initial drawbacks, however, the potential for realizing Herschel's dream continued to interest researchers in Czechoslovakia, other parts of Europe, and in the United States. Modifications were introduced: the lenses were made thinner, and finally a working product emerged. Five years of improvements and clinical-tests were conducted on the lens before the FDA, which termed it a drug, approved it as safe and suitable for its purpose. Their caution, after the thalidomide tragedies of the immediate past, was understandable. Two testing phases were employed: one with laboratory animals to insure the lens's non-toxicity, and one by selected eye practitioners for trials on humans.

Finally, with a great deal of fanfare, approval by the FDA was announced in 1971. The soft lens was then available in the United States, although it had been offered in Europe for several years prior and had created something less than a stir in contact lens fitting circles—for problems later to emerge.

Accompanying the new lenses' utilization for visual purposes, its liquid absorbability suggested its use for certain eye conditions requiring the instillation of drops over a more or less constant period. Approval for this purpose was later received from the FDA and a soft lens, somewhat differently produced, is currently in such use. For this therapy the lens is drenched in antibiotic of choice and releases continuous medication to the infected eye, virtually forming an optical bandage.

Only medium-grade nearsighted prescriptions were obtainable at first—of doubtful optical clarity. Later, farsighted prescriptions were offered, with some optical improvement, and also prescriptions for aphakia. HEMA's fitting was not too dissimilar to that of PMMA lenses although, because of its absorptive characteristics, certain tests requiring tinted fluid were not employed.

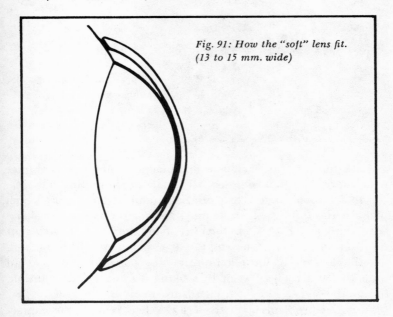

Fig. 91: How the "soft" lens fit.
(13 to 15 mm. wide)

Initial reactions of wearers seemed quite good but some of HEMA's basic defects remained, however, and even to this day present problems.

First, the lens was larger—13 to 15 mm.—than the PMMA lens which was 8 to 9 mm. (Fig. 91) and this accounted for its comfort. But its flexibility made it fit like a glove in some cases, especially with tight lids, and produce the tight lens effect which troubled the very early PMMA wearers. Second, lid movement seemed to distort the lens surface, causing it to ripple or flex with each blink; vision was affected. Third, the aqueous solution in the HEMA caused a hazy appearance, much as the fluid used in early PMMA lenses did. Fourth, the glovelike fit could prevent oxygen from reaching the cornea and this would be a serious impairment. Without this oxygen, gained from the atmosphere (and from the lids in sleep), loss of transparency would result. Other severe effects might follow. Fifth, it was observed that deterioration of the actual HEMA was much faster than of

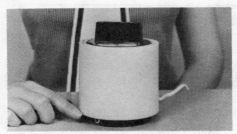

Fig. 92: "Aseptor" used for boiling lenses.

PMMA (p. 181). In fact, one manufacturer did not guarantee it for more than four months: All in all, a discomfiting picture.

And insofar as the bacterial contamination factor which plagued the initial, experimental stages of the Czechoslovakian-born lens, the FDA considered it mandatory that a stringent sterilization procedure be employed—either in the form of boiling the lens daily for ten minutes, for one type utilizing an "Aseptor" unit (Fig. 92) ; or by soaking it in antiseptic solution, for another type. This in itself turned many wearers off.

Current problems with the HEMA lens remind the contact lens fitter of some of the problems encountered with the PMMA fluid-using lens of more than a generation ago. Some researchers have remarked on this resemblance with a sense of *dèjà vu,* and have opined that the HEMA lens is going through the same stage now that the PMMA survived thirty years ago. As a matter of fact, ongoing experiments· are trying to overcome some of HEMA's problems by the use of a rigid central lens section surrounded by a flexible outer section—reminding one of the glass-centered, plastic-surrounded lens of the mid-thirties.

Other experiments involve newer materials, such as the silicone-rubber lens. This does not absorb liquid but simply retains its rubbery state when wet or dry. It is unique in permitting oxygen to go through it. As yet approval by the FDA has not been gained, but, the manufacturer advises, it is expected shortly. Different lenses under experiment also seek this oxygen permeability. FDA approval must be gained on them as well if they ever reach the utilization stage.

But meanwhile the psychological effect of the term "soft" encouraged many would-be contact lens wearers to overcome their fear of applying and removing lenses. And many because of disappointing experience with the soft lens, soon turned to the current PMMA lens with which, as it happens, researchers had overcome the problem of dryness that had, in the first place, impelled the development of HEMA.

Dryness of the surface of the PMMA lens, it had been found, was a major cause of lid sensation and discomfort (p. 149). The underside of the lid being moist naturally, it moved most easily over a moist surface. The water-repelling feature of PMMA was the cause of this dryness and experiments probed its nature: A drop of liquid placed on a solid may spread out to cover the whole surface or it may stay bunched up as a drop. Whether the liquid spreads is decided by the relationship of the forces of cohesion—attraction of the liquid molecules for each other, and adhesion—attraction of the liquid molecules for the solid molecules. The angle between the liquid surface and the solid surface is an indication of the relative values of these forces of adhesion and cohesion. This is known as the angle of contact, and the behavior of a liquid on a solid is spoken of as contact angle (Fig. 93).

This can be measured in degrees of arc and the value obtained

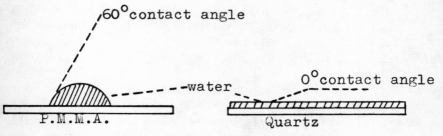

Fig. 93: Contact angles of water on P.M.M.A. (60°) and on quartz surface (.0°)

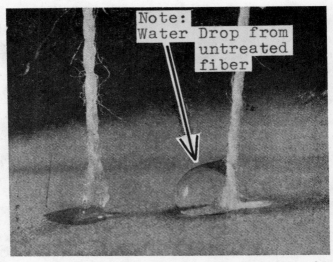

Fig. 93A: Action of a wetting agent, "Polyrad" in treated fiber at left, untreated fiber at right. Magnification x110. (Photographed by Bernard Hoffman, Courtesy Hercules Powder Co.)

is an index of the ability of a liquid to wet a solid. For water and glass (quartz) the angle of contact is 0 degrees—there is complete wetting of the quartz by the water. When the attraction of the liquid for itself is greater than for the solid, there is no wetting; when it is less, there is wetting. Similarly, the reverse is true as well—when the attraction of the solid (molecules) for itself is greater than for the liquid, there is no wetting; when it is less, there is. So with PMMA there is a contact angle of 60° with tears; so it repelled wetting by them. The wetting agents employed to counteract this (Fig. 93A), moreover, proved of limited use.

Once this phenomenon was understood, experiments were undertaken to counteract it. Various substances, transparent all, were fused to the PMMA in order to induce hydrophilia. In the late sixties and early seventies, finally, an ideal substance was found—none other than pure, water-clear inert quartz, the very

THE WALL STREET JOURNAL,
Wednesday, March 10, 1976.

Medical Devices' Regulation by FDA Is Voted by House

By a WALL STREET JOURNAL, *Staff Reporter*

WASHINGTON—The House voted to give the Food and Drug Administration broad new authority to regulate such medical-surgical devices as hearing aids, contact lenses and pacemakers.

The bill is supported by the Ford administration and interested groups. The Senate passed a similar bill last April. Minor differences presumably will be worked out by a conference committee.

Under the bill, all medical devices would have to be registered with the FDA, which could ban any device that poses significant dangers. Some devices would have to meet agency standards regarding construction, testing and labeling. The extent to which a device would be regulated would depend on its importance to health and the potential health hazards from its use. A panel of experts would assist the agency in classifying devices.

New devices would have to be approved by the agency before they could be marketed. Some existing devices, including all devices meant to be implanted in the human body, also would require approval. Makers of such existing devices would have 30 months to seek approval.

The vote to pass the bill was 362 to 32.

same employed in the earliest contact lenses. (Speaking of history repeating itself!) Its bonding to the PMMA surface transferred its 0° contact angle to the surface of the hydrophobic methyl-methacrylate. Thus dryness was eliminated.

Two more years were to elapse before research achieved a molecularly thin coating applied in a vacuum to PMMA's surface. Thickness was one-half to six-tenths of a micron (.0005 to .0006 mm.) so the crucial thinness of the lens (.10 to .25 mm.) was imperceptibly altered. Finally, in early 1974 a patent was granted this process. What was accomplished was the virtual elimination of the dryness which had long plagued the PMMA wearer, even when all the other problems were nonexistent. Friction was gone as the eyelid moved over the lens.

What of the future for flexible lenses, HEMA or otherwise? Far from dim, one might still say. Because the very idea of flexibility or softness, if you will, the concept of a gel-like lens which captured Sir John Herschel's imagination 150 years ago, still promises an attractive, fear-allaying picture to the would-be contact lens wearer. The fear of putting a hard object onto the eye (see Chapter XIV)—that a too forceful impact would be painful and injurious—that a sensation would persist of a foreign body in the eye—this fear would be allayed. Additional research, perhaps in venting the glove-fitting soft lens to achieve better tear and air flow beneath it, as well as making the lens air- and tear-permeable, is a promising direction.

Yet the most attractive lure still remains—to achieve a lens with continuous wear—day-in, day-out, week-in, week-out, even year-in, and year-out. Occasional reports of six months and longer wearing filter in, especially from European sources where untested lenses are worn without restriction. In the U.S. a rare case was reported of a Cleveland man who claims to have worn his lenses (unidentified) continuously for more than five years.

But current professional opinion is definitely against such wearing.

More and more, as new problems arise with recently devised chemical products and their effect on human tissues and health, the prognosis for future, different lenses must be guarded. Not surprisingly, the attention which ophthalmic researchers must pay to these reactions brought into focus another area warranting investigation—that of environmental pollution and atmospheric deterioration which might present a threat to the human eye.

Approximate ranges of wavelengths λ in
vacuum (or air) for the visible and adjacent regions
of the electromagnetic spectrum; 1 A ≡ 10^{-8} cm.

Range	Wavelength range (A)
Near ultraviolet	1600 to 3800
Violet	3800 to 4500
Blue	4500 to 5000
Green	5000 to 5700
Yellow	5700 to 5900
Orange	5900 to 6100
Red	6100 to 7500
Infrared	7500 to 2×10^6 (or 0.02 cm)

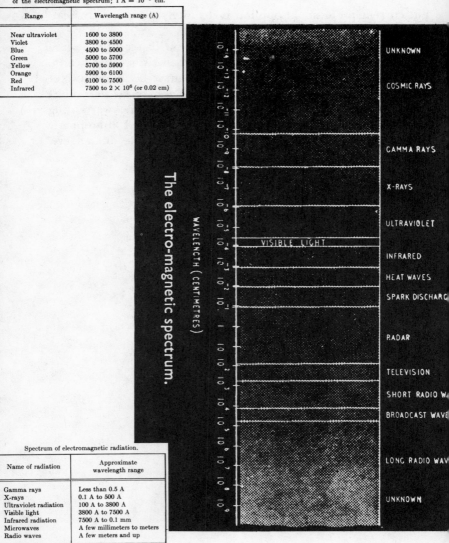

The electro-magnetic spectrum.

Spectrum of electromagnetic radiation.

Name of radiation	Approximate wavelength range
Gamma rays	Less than 0.5 A
X-rays	0.1 A to 500 A
Ultraviolet radiation	100 A to 3800 A
Visible light	3800 A to 7500 A
Infrared radiation	7500 A to 0.1 mm
Microwaves	A few millimeters to meters
Radio waves	A few meters and up

Fig. 94: The electro-magnetic spectrum.

XX

Radiation and the Eye

Life exists and the human eye is a sound, vital organ. As our opening chapter related, millions of years of evolution on earth, subject to the environmental conditions which became what surround us today, have brought humans and their eyes to their present state. Not the least of these is the radiation enveloping the earth—primarily from the earth's star, our sun. Because 50% of the sun's cast-off energy, engendering, fostering, and supporting life on earth, is in the form of visual rays, our eyes developed as they did. Had our evolution taken place on some other planet, farther from or nearer its sun, perhaps one of the Red Dwarf stars, the eyes might have evolved under different radiation and become more responsive to it—infrared most likely. Our perception of objects and the space environment would have been different.

But develop our eyes did . . . no other proof is needed that the radiation reaching the earth today is basically not hostile. Except, we must not forget, that it is filtered by the earth's atmosphere (Figs. 94, 95, 95A). From the Environmental Studies Board of the National Academy of Sciences (Washington, 1973, p. 35):

"An increase in total terrestrial ultraviolet radiation could make this unpleasant injury [conjunctivitis and photophthalmia] more common in the absence of adequate shielding. . . . In addition, ultraviolet radiation has been implicated in the etiology of cataracts. . . ." Researchers at the National Cancer Institute have estimated that 60 to 90% of all cancers are caused by environmental factors, from ultraviolet rays to plastics and pesticides.

Their point is that atmospheric disruption, which impedes filtration of ultraviolet rays, presents a threat to life and the eye. Indeed, the *New York Times* (2/19/76, p. 21) carried an article in which atmospheric scientists concluded that a reversal of the earth's magnetic field 700,000 years ago, coupled with simultaneous solar flares, caused destruction of part of the ozone shield protecting life from ultraviolet radiation. Several species of sea animals became extinct. And they estimated that if solar flares comparable to those of August, 1972 occurred during another such reversal (expected 20 or 30 centuries hence), stratospheric ozone would be reduced by nearly 10% and ground-level ultraviolet damage increased by 15%. It was agreed that any ozone layer weakening would permit strong ultraviolet rays to kill some species of plant and animal life. Evolution of the surviving life might then take another direction. The effect of such weakening may only just be beginning to be felt on life and, in turn, the eye.

The electromagnetic spectrum shows radio waves the longest known and cosmic rays the shortest. Between them there is the range from television, radar, heat and infrared rays to the visible spectrum. Approximately at 770 nanometers (1 nanometer = 1/millionth of a mm. = 10 A.U.) the red rays become visible. Then the orange, yellow, green, blue and violet. At 400 nm. the ultraviolet appears, descending to X rays, to gamma rays and finally to the shortest known—the cosmic rays.

Sir Isaac Newton was the first, in 1672, to experiment with a prism and produce the separation of white light into colors (Fig. 25C). Before this, only rainbows showed the effect. In the 300 years following, fuller understanding has been reached of color and the electromagnetic spectrum. Like visual rays, ultraviolet excites the photochemical receptors of the retina and lead to photophobia, fear of light.

In turn this may lead to destruction or proliferation of the retinal tissues that absorb the rays. Before they reach the retina, absorption takes place in the cornea (below 295 nm.), the lens

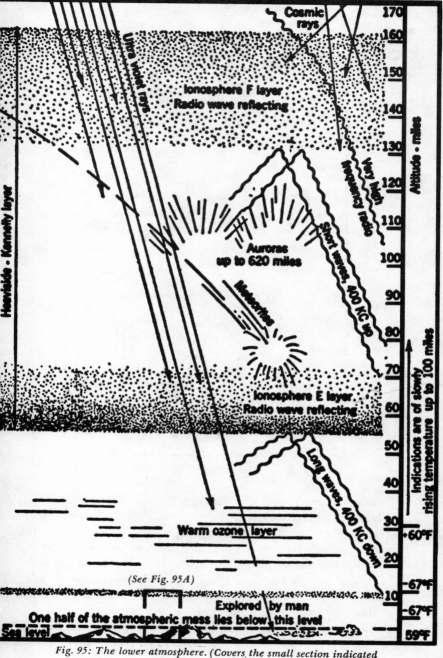

Fig. 95: The lower atmosphere. (Covers the small section indicated in Fig. 95A)

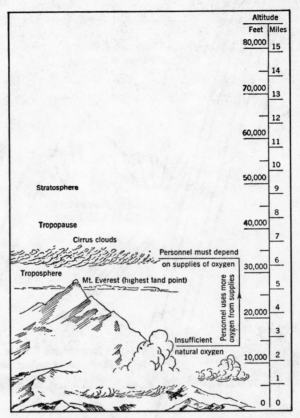

Fig. 95A: Atmosphere below 15 mi. (Detail from Fig. 95)

(below 350 nm.), and the vitreous humour (below 270 nm.) (Fig. 96). Other radiations, shorter ones such as X rays, gamma rays and the particulate radiations of radium and atomic explosions, produce skin and body involvement as well as ocular lesions, but these are primarily laboratory-induced and protected. As indeed are all forms of therapeutic administration of ultraviolet and shorter radiation used to promote healing of indolent or sluggish wounds and for disinfectant purposes or curative measures for rickets and certain skin and lymph node diseases.

The eye can be affected adversely by visible rays as well.

Ordinary light may occasionally be bothersome—glare, etc., but in moderate amounts does no permanent damage. Visual receptors are exhausted, leaving the retina temporarily insensitive. Looking at the sun during an eclipse may cause permanent injury (eclipse blindness) because of the enormous concentration of radiant energy in a very small volume of tissues, producing local heating and subsequent tissue damage.

Radiation from longer wavelengths, infrared and higher, contains too little energy to cause chemical effects—their impact is that of heat and its sequelae. But those of shorter wavelengths contain more energy and do produce effects. Cells may die or be stimulated to cancer-like reproduction. Capillary paralysis and engorgement may result, and outpouring of serum may be characteristic. Corneal absorption may show effects of nuclear fragmentation "similar to that of mustard gas." One ophthalmologist likens it to "a city after a hit and miss bombing attack . . . some epithelial cells are destroyed while others remain unaffected . . . there are 'hits' by the ionizing radiation destroying certain groups of cells." But no permanent damage generally results except that the tissue is hypersensitive to light for a long time thereafter.

In the lens, coagulation of lens protein and the formation of opacities could follow. Its permeability is changed and its auto-oxidation system diminished. Like the cornea, the lens is without blood vessels, but without exposure to atmospheric oxygen, depends entirely on osmosis for oxygen and nutrients. Curtailment of this could cause cataract; that this affliction is common in tropical countries like India would indicate the culpability of excessive radiation. Vitreous absorption (below 270 nm.) has hardly been researched because this wavelength does not pass the cornea. The retina absorbs all rays down to 350 nm. and, without the lens, to 295.

Ultraviolet absorption by the atmosphere is almost entirely achieved by its ozone—an oxygen derivative formed by electrostatic discharge. Since oxygen composes approximately 23% of the atmosphere, it is a fertile source and, being subject to electrostatic forces surrounding the earth, forms ozone plentifully. Ozone absorption of the ultraviolet strips the rays of their energy

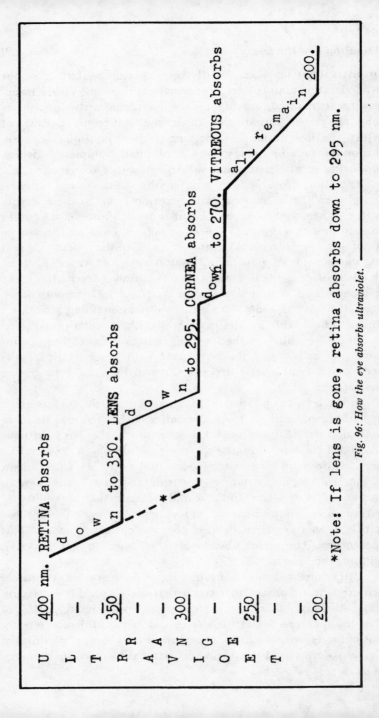

Fig. 96: How the eye absorbs ultraviolet.

—thus the earth's surface is effectively shielded from excessive ultraviolet penetration.

For several years now, scientists have felt that emissions of various chemicals have been denuding the ozone and, to some extent, the oxygen source as well. High-level emission of nitrogen oxides by jet planes, it is claimed, also causes this stripping and the current controversy concerning the Concorde SST revolves in good measure around this threat. Certain chemicals on earth, aerosol spray, for one, have been charged with aggravating the problem. Hard evidence is yet to be gained that the ozone layers have been depleted in recent years, despite such high-level flights and widespread aerosol use. At least one study suggests that ozone thickness actually increased during the sixties. Theoretically, of course, the possibility cannot be dismissed. Results of a thinned ozone layer would be so devastating as to warrant every precaution.

This was the background when contact lens researchers turned to new plastics or variations of old ones to overcome HEMA difficulties. Years before, in the mid-sixties, during research to solve the dryness PMMA problem, there was minute and painstaking experimentation with PMMA itself. The fact was uncovered that there was a color variation of PMMA claimed to be ultraviolet-filtering. Only this color, a shade of yellowish-amber, had this property and the manufacturer's spectrographic analyses supported the assertion.

However, whether the same quality would be retained after grinding the plexiglass down from the manufacturer's testing thicknesses of .060″ to 1″ (slightly thinner than 2mm. to 25mm.) to the contact lens thinness of 1/10th mm. to ¼ mm. was the question. Tests were made on lenses of these thinnesses over half a dozen years. Results were encouraging. Spectrophotometric readings showed ultraviolet opacity down to 1 or 2 percent in all wavelengths. Clinical and use tests with actual wearers— skiers, flyers, sunbathers—showed almost complete glare elimination. Not until the early seventies, when the quartz-coating process was evolved and adopted, were experiments refined to ascertain the effect of the quartz additive. Borne in mind was the fact that quartz, the common ingredient of ordinary glass

Laboratory Analysis No. 32360

Ultraviolet Transmittance

Through Contact Lens	@ 400 nanometers 0 %	Descending to 0 % @ 330nm.	(2% @ 280 nm.*)
PMMA Experimental			
Brown	44	10 @ 330nm.	
Blue	69	0 @ 320	(8.5 @ 273)
Green	52	0 @ 320	(8.0 @ 275)
Smoke	52	0 @ 245	(11 @ 315-05, 13.5 @ **265**)
Clear Uncoated	31	0 @ 325	(4.0 @ 273)
HEMA Clear	**36**	0 @ 240	
Tints not produced	—	1	
Eyeglass Lens			
Plastic	83	0 @ 270	
Glass	38	0 @ 350	
Ray-Ban	51	0 @ 330	
Photo-Gray	51	0 @ 330	
Pure Quartz	38	0 @ 350	

*Note. "The 2% transmittance...@ the 280 nm. region might well be undetected by a less sensitive instrument than the DK 2-A".

Fig. 97: Chart of Ultraviolet Transmittance.

and eyeglasses, was already known to be opaque to ultraviolet radiation below 350 nm.

Results were positive. Reflection from snow and water was less bothersome; the quartz seemed to enhance the filtering quality. Spectrophotometric tests were taken in late '75 and early '76, this time with newly improved, highly sensitive instruments. In the words of the analytical laboratory, the lenses submitted were "measured through an aperture slightly smaller than the diameter of the lens with *sample* and *reference* paths calibrated to 100% transmittance and zero transmittance using a Beckman Model DK 2-A ratio recording Spectrophotometer. Spectacle lenses were measured in a similar fashion except areas corresponded to normal optics of the DK 2A."

Twelve samples were checked: seven of contact lenses, six PMMA and one HEMA; four of spectacle lenses, one of plastic and three of glass; and the quartz additive (Fig. 97).

The experimental lens "exhibited a maximum percent transmittance of 2% at 280 nanometers. All wavelengths from 400 to 290 nm. and from 270 to 220 nm. were essentially zero percent transmittance." The others ranged from 31% to 69% transmittance at 400 nm. for the PMMA lenses; at 36% for the HEMA lens; at 83% for the plastic eyeglass lens and 38% for the glass eyeglass lens, with the latter's zero transmittance below 350 nm.; to 51% transmittance for the sunglasses at 400 nm. and zero below 330 nm. Pure quartz tested the same as glass and its zero transmittance below 350 nm. appeared to reinforce the experimental lens' opacity in these wavelengths.

The findings of the investigators and the reports of wearers were confirmed. An unexpected bonus was offered the PMMA wearer—a lens guarding the eye from radiation which, pathogenic already, might cause more damage if the warnings of environmental protectionists and atmospheric scientists were not heeded. Odd that this almost science-fictional eye protection was uncovered during rather prosaic research on a routine health aid, glamorous though the contact lens might be. Perhaps the future would require just such a protective shield over portions of the earth where life might be threatened by penetrating ultraviolet.

But what the future may bring is what we turn to now. . . .

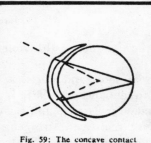

Fig. 59: The concave contact lens has a flatter outside curve than the corneal surface.

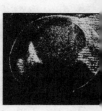

CONTACT LENSES ... The Firs

1887	1936	1945	1950
ALL–GLASS SCLERAL	GLASS–PLASTIC SCLERAL	ALL–PLASTIC (PMMA*)SCLERAL	CORNEA PMMA
<u>Breakable</u>	Breakable	~~Breakable~~	~~Breakab~~
<u>Fluid-using</u>	Fluid-using	Fluid-using	~~Fluid-u~~
		<u>Psycho. Resis.</u>	Psych. R
			<u>Lid Sens</u>
			<u>Dryness</u>

(Underlining _____
  indicates first appearance)

           *Poly Methyl Meth Acrylate (Hydrophobic)

       **Hydroxy Ethyl Meth Acrylate (Hydrophilic)
       ((Classifed as a drug needing FDA approval))

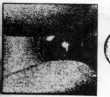

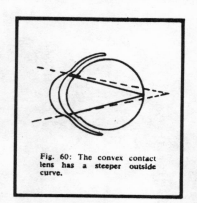

Fig. 60: The convex contact lens has a steeper outside curve.

One-Hundred Years

1960		1974	1976	2076
VENTED PMMA		COATED PMMA	UV-FILTER PMMA	?
	1971 "SOFT" HEMA**			
Breakable	Breakable	Breakable	Breakable	
Fluid-use	Fluid-use	Fluid-use	Fluid-use	
Psy. Re.	Psy. Re.(?)	Psych.Re.	Psych. Res.	
Lid-Sen.	Lid-Sens.	Lid-Sen.	Lid-Sense.	
Dryness	Dryness	Dryness	Dryness	
U.V.Tran.	U.V.Tran.	U.V.Tran.	U.V.-Trans.	
	Limited Rx			
	Cloudiness			
	Deteriora.			
	Contamina.(?)			

245

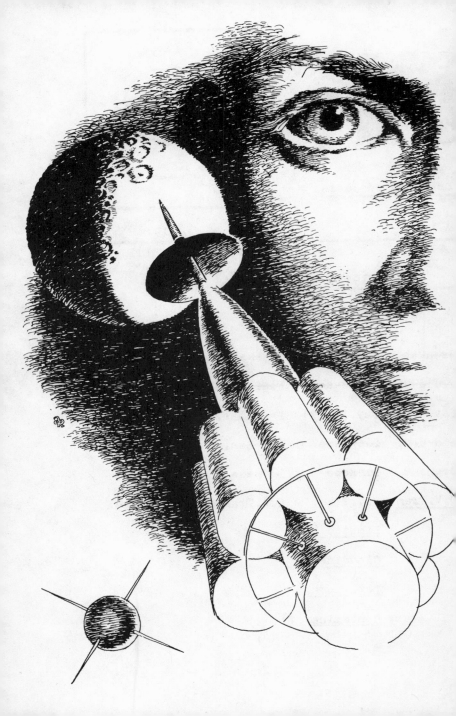

XXI
The Next Hundred Years

It's been said that the past century saw more advances than the preceding fifty. . . . The next one is bound to exceed it.

Back in 1962, barely a year after laser itself was first produced (Union Carbide Corp., 9/17/61), it was noticed that a laser beam showed a speckle pattern when it was reflected. A farsighted person observing this while moving his head detected it moving in the same direction; a near-sighted one oppositely. Now, using a rotating drum with this laser reflection, it is possible for astigmatism as well to be detected and even measured. The procedure is fast becoming a viable clinical one.

The direct employment of visible radiation, either in the form of laser or finely focused beams of intense light, has been shown to cause minute burns on the retina. Infrared rays may do this as well. The photocoagulation resulting will destroy abnormal blood vessels which lead to serious loss of vision. These are produced in certain ocular diseases or by systemic abnormalities affecting the eye. Today the laser beam, in particular, is almost routinely used; by "spot-welding" detached retinas (95% success) it seals off the hemorrhages and proliferating blood vessels in the eyes of thousands of diabetics.

Utilizing a weak laser beam for accurate measurement of the critical flow of blood and oxygen in the living retina, without touching the patient, has been recently devised.

Corneal transplants are being carried out by thousands in every part of the world. Research has developed practical methods for storing and transporting eye tissues. Modern surgical techniques fit pre-cut and premeasured discs of donated corneal tissue exactly to areas where damaged tissue has been excised. When human tissue cannot be transplanted, clear plastic buttons have been devised which may be fastened permanently into a small hole in the corneal surface.

In many countries, particularly the developing ones where advanced surgical methods are not readily available or where scarcity of donors is a problem, contact lenses have emerged as devices of choice for corneal replacement, scars and low visual acuity. "All patients with corneal scarring should be treated with contact lenses, especially in the four following cases: a) where surgery can be avoided by fitting the eye with a contact lens; b) in pre-operative assessment of retinal functions as a guide for visual prognosis; c) to visualize the fundus in scarred and conical corneas; and d) to improve visual acuity in post-operative regular or irregular astigmatism following keratoplasty (corneal transplant)." (Dr. R. Frasad Centre for Ophthalmic Sciences, All India Institute of Medical Sciences, New Delhi, 1975).

There are 400,000 cataract operations performed each year in the United States with 98% success. Today, the lens is reached through a tiny incision, removed by freezing techniques or emulsified by ultrasound, and siphoned out through the same instrument. New drugs prevent post-operative infections. The next day the patient is out of bed and in a few days is home without extraordinary restrictions on his movements. Formerly immobilization for days or weeks was necessary. The implantation of plastic lenses—termed "intra-ocular"—to replace the removed cataractous lens of the eye is becoming increasingly routine, particularly in the case of elderly patients. (See Fig. 38.)

A new surgical procedure, vitrectomy, already has restored the sight of some who were blind for years from blood hemorrhaging into the normally clear vitreous, the gel-like substance between the lens and the retina. Research has developed a new surgical instrument permitting entry into the center of the eye through a very small incision. Used under the operating micro-

NEW DEVICE SENDS LIGHT A LONG WAY

Union Carbide Unit 'Growing' Crystal That Beams Data

By WILLIAM M. FREEMAN

Crystals that can send beams of light across distances as great as a million miles are being "grown" on a production basis by the crystal products department of Linde Company, a division of the Union Carbide Corporation.

Such a crystal, a composite material synthesis of rubies and other gems.

The latest effect—in the laser, the maser and the iraser, among other variations—is to concentrate light so intensely that it becomes "coherent." In this state, light can carry information that may be used to direct manufacturing operations and perhaps perform other tasks that are now only in the theoretical stage.

The achievement of concentrating light into a beam far brighter than that from the sun, thus producing heat such as the sun might produce if its light were to be so concentrated, holds rich promise for the future.

With the radio wave area crowded, and microwaves getting to be crowded, too, the infra-red and visible light spectra represent a great new highway of the future for communications.

THE NEW YORK TIMES,
Sunday, September 17, 1961.

THE NEW YORK TIMES, Friday, April 2, 1976.

Light Beam Treatments Reduce Diabetic Blindness

By HAROLD M. SCHMECK Jr.

Special to The New York Times

WASHINGTON, April 1—Evidence that a treatment called photocoagulation reduces the risk of blindness in some diabetes patients was made public today by the National Institutes of Health.

Dr. Carl Kupfer, director of the National Eye Institute, a unit of the N.I.H., described the evidence as conclusive. The study, still in progress, involves about 1,720 patients and 16 major hospitals and research institutions.

The results made public today indicate that treatment by photocoagulation reduces by more than half the risk of blindness in eyes seriously threatened by the condition called diabetic retinopathy.

Diabetic retinopathy is among the leading causes of blindness in the United States. The National Eye Institute estimates that there are more than 300,000 persons whose sight is threatened by the condition. Its underlying cause is unknown, but the chance of its ment of the other eye is being considered for the patients who have already had treatment in one eye. The decision is to be made on an individual basis, depending on the particular patient's condition.

The treatment is by no means a panacea, said Dr. Matthew D. Davis, of the University of Wisconsin Medical School. He is chairman of the diabetic retinopathy study executive committee. The physician said the treatment was not always effective, had some drawbacks and did not offer a cure of the underlying biological problem.

Nevertheless, Dr. Davis said, a substantially larger number of untreated eyes were lost to the disease. The report said 16.3 percent of the untreated eyes followed for two years or more went blind while only 6.4 percent of treated eyes did so.

In some cases, persons whose eyes were treated lost some degree of visual acuity or some peripheral vision, but these scope, the device safely cuts away vitreous strands, chops them up and siphons them out through its hollow needle, at the same time replacing the vitreous with a clear fluid. The most rapidly increasing cause of blindness in the United States, diabetic resinopathy, is on the list to be considered for this treatment.

Ocular drug treatment is progressing phenomenally. For example, control of devastating Herpes viruses, an acute inflammation of the lids, and conjunctiva, and a major cause of corneal blindness, by a new drug has just been announced. (Research to Prevent Blindness, New York, 1976). In the success of this drug may also be found an answer to Herpes genital infections, the nation's most prevalent and incurable form of venereal disease. Another new drug is demonstrating its effectiveness in controlling numerous cases of previously intractable glaucoma.

And, in the case of glaucoma, its early detection has been found to be most decisive. The recently announced NCT (noncontact) tonometer, advancing the instrument used in glaucoma detection to a non-touching of the cornea stage, is a major step forward. This should help glaucoma-testing become an integral part of every eye examination.

The phoropter (Fig. 35B) of the thirties has been computerized. Now it can serve as another retinoscope, p. 64, formerly the only objective refracting means. Infrared light and a photo-detector find the eye's focal point in seconds. A print-out of the correcting prescription follows.

Adapted to ophthalmoscopy (p. 63), a red-free filter is permitting thorough study of different retinal layers. Red light is refracted less than green (Fig. 25C). In a normal eye the red focuses behind the retina, the green before it, (Fig. 98). For years this fact was used to refine presbyopic lenses as well as myopic and hyperopic. Filtering out the red rays, which penetrated the deeper retinal layers, permitted the yellow-green to be reflected at the top layer. This allows the examiner to view the nerve fibers which lie there. And their pattern in health or disease can be analyzed (Fig. 99).

In addition, sharp contrast is allowed between blood vessels or hemorrhages and the retinal background because hemoglobin

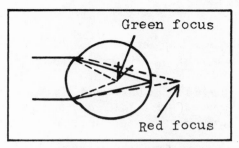

Fig. 98: The focus of red and green light in normal eye. (Highly exaggerated) Myopic eye sees better in red; hyperopic in green.

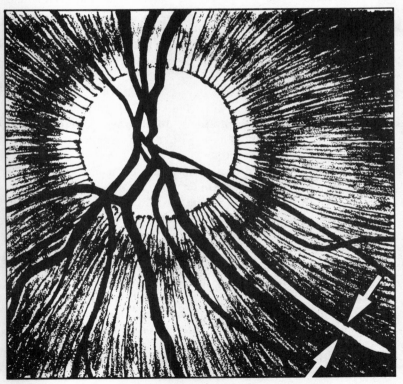

Fig. 99: Nerve fiber bundle defect between arrows. (Courtesy, T.M. Wiley, O.D.)

transmits the red and absorbs the shorter wavelengths. Red filtering highlights them. This aids in detecting and diagnosing systemic conditions which have ocular manifestations.

Refinements in the use of pin-hole discs (p. 118) to improve vision for the near-blind, now termed "low-vision" patients, are frequent. Sharper sight in addition to an increased field is obtained.

High-powered concave contact lenses as oculars in telescopic spectacles (p. 179) are more in use today. Only regular spectacles with high-powered convex lenses need be worn over them to achieve the telescopic effect. A far greater visual field is gained; restricted movement is overcome and a more normal appearance presented. A stronger eyeglass lens, even a bifocal, limited only by grinding problems, will permit near vision. With a high-powered convex contact lens as the ocular, the microscopic spectacle also has been bettered.

Higher or lower lighting levels as aids to low vision are becoming more understood: patients with glaucoma, aphakia, pathological myopia with pin-point pupils, these function better with high illumination. Those with albinism, aniridia, central corneal or lens opacities, prefer minimum illumination.

New types of magnifiers, near-point telescopes, monocular and binocular magnifiers, cylinder and absorbent loupes, minifiers, comparators,—the list is endless—all these have passed beyond drawing boards. A multiple-lens magnifier affords flexibility with peripheral color control, ranging from magnification of 20 diopters to as high as 100. The normal size of an object is its size when viewed at 2 diopters or 20 inches; so viewing it clearly at 10x nearer, 2 inches from the eye, magnifies it enormously.

Conceived and developed in close coordination with the U.S. Government's Night Vision Laboratories, electronic binoculars have been introduced by the International Telephone & Telegraph Corp. (Fig. 100). These help in the incipient night-blindness stage of an insidious retinal disease called "retinitis pigmentosa." This afflicts more than 100,000 United States residents who, little by little, will go totally blind.

Meanwhile the electronic binoculars detect light even in

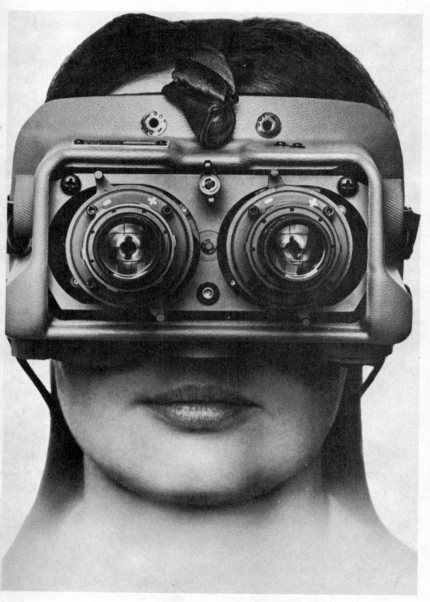

Fig. 100. The Electronic Binoculars by I.T.T.
(Courtesy I.T.T. Corp.)

near-total darkness—then electronically magnify it so that even failing eyes can see. Less expensive, pocket-sized models are currently in work with the National Retinitis Pigmentosa Foundation so that more children and adults, who become afflicted each day and need them, can have them.

Closed circuit television is fast becoming a revolutionary visual aid. Passing easily from sports and entertainment viewing, high angular and zoom magnification together with contrast control make it ideal for low-vision aid. Adding close-up lenses in the lens system enhances magnification. TV's expanding use in education will certainly encourage further visual correction and normalization.

A significant variation of the electronic imagery already detailed, is the reported use of ultrasonic sound waves broadcast in a blind or low-visioned person's environment from a transmitter built into the front of his spectacles. Echoes are picked up by receivers mounted in the spectacle temples on each side of the wearer's head. The difference in loudness, pitch, and tuning can help users locate the source of the echoes in space. This resembles the squeak made by a bat where returning echoes guide its movements. Experiments are well under way, it is reported, to give the visually handicapped the perception of objects around him by their characteristic sounds—a virtual "sound picture" of his environment.

Other research concerns migraine headaches and vague feelings of eyestrain routinely associated with ocular symptoms. What is their amenability to acupuncture rather than refractive correction? The question is open. The whole subject of diet therapy for ocular as well as systemic ills is receiving renewed attention. Where it will lead is highly promising.

And what of eyes in space? It is granted that when man is called upon to survive in extremely exotic conditions such as fast aircraft, space vehicles or adrift in space, he must augment his sensory system with man-made aids—electronic devices such as radar, for an elementary first. But close-up photographs of the moon add not nearly as much to human knowledge as the actual stepping of man on its surface. There, on-the-spot exploration, with experiments spontaneously improvised and all his senses employed, is undoubtedly the most rewarding. The ambiguity of what is above and what is below in the weightless state is only one indication of the physiological imbalances which occur in outer space. The visual impact of this disorientation, its resultant confusion, distortion, and optical illusion, are still to be understood.

Gravitational and radiation effects on intraocular fluids and pressure, on the eye's nutrition, on its tissues, cells and blood vessels, are being explored and classified. Countermeasures are being tested. Aerospace medicine's research in these directions is well on its way. Today.

So it goes on, advance crowding advance. Over thousands of years, it is possible that the lessened atmospheric filtering of ultraviolet rays may necessitate the eyes' adaptation for survival. Evolution will continue. Our sun's aging may bring it into the red dwarf category with most of its radiations in the infrared range. The eye may well adapt to see infrared—its increasing tendency to myopia with resulting better vision under red light, already noted, seems a step in that direction. But that is the far-distant future.

In today's world, we witness many of the dreams of a mere fifteen years ago becoming realities. In the diagnosis of eye diseases, one ophthalmologist puts it, "We are experiencing a technical explosion. Fluorescein photography, ultrasound, optic disc mapping, 180-degree retinal observation—a listing would fill pages. We observe ongoing processes of this magnificent, complex organ invisible just fifteen years ago and undreamed of fifty years ago."

If imaginative research continues at its present pace, advances of the next fifteen years will surely surpass those of the past hundred.